GERIATRICS

Guidelines in Medicine

VOLUME 1

GERIATRICS

A.N.Exton-Smith
MD, FRCP

Barlow Professor of Geriatric Medicine, University College Hospital Medical School, London

and P. W. Overstall
MB, MRCP

Consultant in Geriatric Medicine, University College Hospital, London

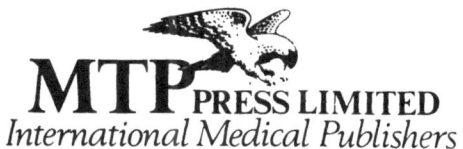
MTP PRESS LIMITED
International Medical Publishers

Published by
MTP Press Limited
Falcon House
Lancaster, England

British Library Cataloguing in Publication Data

Exton-Smith, Arthur Norman
    Geriatrics. – (Guidelines in medicine; vol. 1).
    1. Geriatrics
    I. Title
    II. Overstall, P W III. Series
    618.9'7   RC952

ISBN-13: 978-94-011-7193-9   e-ISBN-13: 978-94-011-7191-5
DOI: 10.1007/978-94-011-7191-5

Contents

ACKNOWLEDGEMENTS

We wish to thank our secretaries, Judith Calver and Kathleen Trew, Mr V. K. Asta, medical artist, and Mr A. C. J. Lees, medical photographer at the Medical School.

1
Ageing

The more one thinks and talks about 'the elderly' the easier it is to forget that in clinical practice one is always dealing with an individual. Although some useful generalizations may be made about the ageing process and the differences in disease presentation and management of the older patient, it is a mistake to regard the elderly as a homogeneous group. Indeed, variations between individuals tend to increase with age.

The physiological, psychological and social changes that occur in old age can be regarded as being, potentially, an experience common to all and comparable to the effect of puberty on adolescents. How an individual responds to growing old appears to depend more upon his previous pattern of life than upon anything in the ageing process itself.

LIFE EXPECTANCY

This is a statistical projection based on the annual death rate and is not related to ageing changes in individuals. A simple formula was shown by Gompertz in 1825 to predict accurately the probability of dying at any given age: the probability rising exponentially with

1

increasing age beyond 30 years.

There has been a remarkable increase in life expectancy in developed countries over the last century. This has been largely due to improvements in nutrition and public health measures which reduced water- and food-borne diseases. The influence of immunization and therapy had little effect on mortality until the introduction of sulphonamides in 1935, and even since then has probably remained much less important than continued improvements in nutrition and the environment (McKeown, 1976).

Despite the considerable reduction in deaths occurring before the age of 65 there has been very little increase in life expectancy for those who reach that age, so that although life expectancy at birth between 1911 and now has increased from 49 to 70 years for men and from 52 to 76 years for women, there has been only a 1-year increase in life expectancy for men at 65 years, and 4 years for women. The population 'bulge' of elderly people is due to late Victorian and Edwardian fecundity. Large families, that were raised in the expectation that half would die in infancy, have in fact survived. It is not so much that the elderly are living longer as that more are reaching old age.

THEORIES OF AGEING

There is at present no single theory that adequately explains ageing throughout the body. A satisfactory model for ageing in connective tissue does not explain changes in epithelial cells that divide throughout life, or non-dividing cells such as neurones. Indeed it is probable that different tissues age in different ways.

Genetic factors

Genetic factors undoubtedly affect ageing, and this is most apparent in variations in life span between different species. Man may live for 70 years, but a butterfly for only 24 hours. Within the same species the range of individual life spans is smaller than that between different species, and it was shown in the 1930s that the life span of any human

2

could be predicted with some accuracy given the age at death of the parents and four grandparents. The question is whether genetic material is programmed from the start to produce ageing after a certain period (in the same way that puberty is triggered) or whether genetic instability, either through copying errors or through chromosomal damage, produces malfunction.

Error accumulation

Actively dividing cells depend on the accurate transmission of genetic material from parent to daughter cell. Information is programmed in nuclear DNA and transcribed to the messenger RNA of the daughter cell, which acts as a template for protein synthesis. Enzymes· are involved at all stages and, if faulty, would impair protein production; eventually the accumulation of errors could cause cell malfunction.

What is not clear though is the cause of the first error. It may be a mutation of nuclear DNA or, just as likely, a failure of feedback mechanisms to correct errors that are inevitable in a biological system. A single faulty enzyme could rapidly produce third- and fourth-generation errors in protein synthesis so that the number of errors needed to impair cell function need only be small. Why this process is not harmful in youth may be due to an efficient immune system that declines with age. Although chromosomal aberrations increase with age it still has to be shown that irreparable faults in DNA, RNA or protein synthesis are the actual cause of ageing.

Mutation

This is defined as a faulty transcription of DNA during mitosis. Ageing may be due to an accumulation of mutations caused by radiation and other environmental hazards such as toxic chemicals. Certainly, repeated small doses of radiation will reduce an animal's life span and the effect of both ageing and radiation is to increase the number of mutations. The longevity of an old animal is inversely proportional to the number of mutations that develop, but there appears to be a fundamental difference between the mutations produced by age and those that follow radiation. For a given number of mutations the life-shortening effect of the naturally produced variety is much

3

greater than that of radiation. In addition, mutations produced by radiation only survive a few divisions and then disappear, which implies that radiation damage is normally repaired (Busse, 1977).

Programmed ageing

The idea that ageing is due to the running down of a biological 'clock' is an attractive one. Growth and puberty are genetically determined and it is probable that ageing is too. For some time it was thought that ageing occurred at a supracellular level in the animal as a whole, since an early *in vitro* experiment had apparently shown that cells could be cultured indefinitely. Immortal cell lines are still cultured (such as the Hela-cell derived from a human cervical carcinoma), but it is now clear that only abnormal cells behave in this way. Hayflick (1976) has shown that there is a fixed number of divisions that a normal cell can undergo before it dies. Normal human embryonic fibroblasts will undergo 50 ± 10 doublings *in vitro*. The *in vitro* doubling capacity declines with increasing age of the animal so that fibroblasts from adults divide only 20 ± 10 times. Predictably, cells grown from patients with progeria, who have accelerated ageing, show a considerable reduction in doubling capacity compared with normal persons of the same age. Hayflick has also shown that the 'clock' controlling the finite number of cell doublings is located in the nucleus, and that although cells may be stored almost indefinitely at low temperatures, when reconstituted the culture will still die after making its total of about 50 doublings.

Cross-linkage

This is an age-related process that is found in collagen, but not in intracellular protein. With age, ester bonds form between collagen molecules producing dense knots that alter the structure and function of connective tissue (Hall, 1976). Skin loses its elasticity, the resilience of intervertebral discs declines, and tendons and collagenous sheaths around muscles become increasingly rigid.

Free radicals

These are molecular fragments which contain an unpaired electron,

4

and are therefore highly reactive. They are formed during normal metabolism and also from chemicals found in food and tobacco. They are considered harmful because it is thought that they increase mutation, promote cross-linkage and may be involved in the development of ageing pigment. Free radicals are inactivated by anti-oxidants, of which Vitamin E is an example. Attempts to show that Vitamin E can prolong life have not yet proved conclusive.

Immune theory

Considerable interest has been shown in the thymus since it may, through its role in maintaining immunological competence, be responsible for the appearance of senescence. If ageing is due to increasing autoimmune aggressiveness it would fit well with the observed age-related involution of the thymus and weakening of immunological surveillance. With advancing age there is a reduction in peripheral blood T-cells, which are responsible for cellular immunity and delayed-type hypersensitivity. Skin-test antigens such as tuberculin and dinitrochlorobenzene (DNCB), which provoke a delayed-type hypersensitivity reaction, are less likely in the elderly to produce a positive result. The decline in T-cells is also associated with a rising incidence of infections and malignancies. B-lymphocytes, which develop into plasma cells and are responsible for the synthesis of circulating antibodies, increase with age. Autoantibodies and serum immunoglobulins (mainly IgG) progressively rise, and so does the incidence of multiple myeloma and giant cell arteritis.

SOCIOLOGICAL FACTORS

Nearly 20% of the population of Great Britain is over the age of 60. This proportion is very similar to that found in France and West Germany and is slightly higher than that in the USA and the Netherlands. India and Brazil have only 4% of the population over 60 years. The

5

majority of the elderly in this country are the 'young old', below the age of 75, who are usually still in good physical and mental health. But this leaves 25% over 75 years; 2.75 million people, who, as a group, are the largest users of Health and Social Services. It is in this group that a considerable increase is expected over the next 20 years.

There is no reason why the projected population figures should cause despair, since in all the industrialized countries affected there already exists the knowledge and skill necessary to maintain an effective service, provided that resources are shifted to meet the new need. More money alone, however, is not sufficient; we need to question some of the widespread assumptions that are made about the elderly.

Negative attitudes

Employment
Most Western countries have a strong work ethos, and prize productivity and earning capacity, so that the retired worker tends to be regarded as a less than useful citizen. The increasing cost of contributions by the working population to maintain adequate pensions for the retired can produce resentment if it is forgotten that much of today's affluence is the fruit of earlier generations' toil. The decline of crafts and family businesses in favour of mechanization and large industrial complexes lessens the value of the older person's experience and often makes his skills obsolete.

Fear of ageing
Each of us must face the prospect of growing old and dying, and the current taboo which surrounds death does not encourage a calm acceptance of the realities. Personal fears of disability and suffering may sometimes be relieved only by adopting denigratory attitudes to the elderly, or by a tendency to sentimentalize. Calling old people 'those geriatrics' or regarding them as naughty children to be patronized by the use of endearments are common examples.

Illness and morale
A common fallacy is to regard all old people as being in poor mental

6

and physical health and as 'blocking' hospital beds up and down the country. In fact 95% of the elderly live in their own homes and most rate their health as good or fair. It is often thought that old people feel sorry for themselves and are bad-tempered, but there is little or no sign of a significant decline in happiness or life satisfaction with age (Palmore and Maddox, 1977).

Sexual experience
The taboo on sex in old age, which survives despite the greater liberality and frankness with which the subject is treated in other age groups, means that difficulties can arise. Kinsey first showed that a large number of the elderly engaged in sexual activity. In the longitudinal study at Duke University it was found that over a 10-year period the percentage of healthy men who had regular sexual intercourse declined from 70% to 25%, but the percentage who retained a sexual interest remained constant at about 80%. In women only 20% reported having regular sexual intercourse and about a third continuing sexual interest, but these percentages remained constant over the 10-year period (Pfeiffer, 1977).

The status of the elderly in our society varies so widely with sex, socioeconomic group and ethnic origin that one should regard with some caution the tendency to ascribe qualities, often negative, to the group as a whole. Constantly emphasizing that the elderly are poor and deprived tends to encourage people to expect the worst. To limit one's concern to purely financial matters may be an implicit denial of the old person's personal and emotional needs (BASW Working Party, 1977).

Poverty

There are substantial differences in income between different retired households, although inequalities are less than in the general population (Age Concern Research Unit, 1977). In 1975 the average weekly income of a household where the head was retired was £34.63, compared with £84.31 for a household where the head was still working.

However, only one retired household in eight has a weekly income close to this average: 37% have weekly incomes below £20, and 13% have incomes of at least £60. By contrast figures for average income per head show that even in the poorest elderly household the income is at least 80% of the average found in households where the head is still working.

As might be expected most elderly households rely heavily on social security benefits, and these payments range from a minimum of 45% to 60% of total average income. Yet when elderly people were asked: 'How much extra money, if any, would you say you and members of your household need to come in each week in order to live without money worries and in health and comfort?' 40% said none, compared with 29% of young adults who replied similarly. The extra money that was needed by the elderly was very small: an average of £8.50 a week, which was less than half the extra amount that young adults felt they needed.

Standard of living

The elderly have a lower rate of ownership of consumer durables than young adults, but are also less likely to have feelings of deprivation (Age Concern Research Unit, 1977). Indeed there is a considerable contrast in the elderly between their standard of living as measured by ownership of consumer goods and how they see it themselves. They generally express much more satisfaction with their standard of living than younger groups. Most elderly people express more satisfaction with their housing, the district they live in, their standard of living and their leisure activities than younger adults. Only in their satisfaction with their health is the trend reversed. The most common complaint in the elderly (25% of the sample) is general aches and pains. Despite the high overall life satisfaction of the elderly, one in five express a very low level of satisfaction. This minority contains a high proportion of women living alone, who regard themselves as being in very poor health.

8

Ageing

Loss

Ageing has been described as a time of loss. The increasing prevalence of suicide and depressive illnesses shows that not all elderly people make a satisfactory adjustment.

Work

Compulsory retirement means not only the loss of a job, but also loss of a routine, comradeship, status and income. For many men, going to

TABLE 1
POINTERS TOWARDS SUCCESSFUL RETIREMENT

---

1 *Plan ahead*
Consider finance, part time job, new routine.

2 *Move house?*
Advantages in moving to smaller house in same district.
Disadvantages of 'the cottage by the sea' (loss of friends and neighbours, isolation, lack of transport, overstretched social services)

3 *Maintain physical activity*
Regular exercise (raise pulse rate to 120/min for 2 min a day and put every joint through a full range of movement). Develop hobbies and games.

4 *Keep up morale*
Maintain mental activity. Question long held beliefs (e.g. political). Make new friends.

5 *Improve home safety*
Check stair rods, remove high shelves and trailing wires.

6 *Find new role*
Remain 'engaged'.

7 *Forget chronological age*

9

work has been the focus of their lives, and some never manage to fill the emptiness that retirement brings. Pre-retirement counselling can produce useful adjustments in attitudes as well as in more practical arrangements. Retirement no longer signals the end of a person's useful life: most who reach retirement age can expect to live for another 15–20 years.

For a woman retirement is often easier because she still has a house to run and usually has developed a network of friends, neighbours, shopkeepers and delivery men around where she lives. However there may be considerable stress on a marriage when husband and wife suddenly find themselves at home together all day.

Gift relationship

The loss of income on retirement threatens the loss of what anthropologists call the gift relationship. Giving money in exchange for goods; labour in return for wages is a fundamental part of life. The ability to 'pay one's way' may be lost either through poverty or disability, and to go from a position of being able to give to that of being only able to receive is, for some, a bitter experience.

Independence

Increasing ill health threatens old people's independence so that many are able to survive at home only with the help of a relative or social services. Physical infirmities may mean that dressing, washing or walking become so troublesome that the person, without being depressed, declares that life has become too difficult and tiring, and that they are ready to die.

Bereavement

Death of spouse, relatives and friends are yet further blows. Grief and even anger need to be worked through, and the person needs help to face the loss and make the necessary adjustments.

Ageing

The mental adjustments of old age are part of the continuous adaptation that goes on throughout life. Despite the similarity of the process at different ages there is an artificial division so that childhood and youth are seen as the time for education; middle age as the period when one builds a career; but it is not usual to recognize old age as a time for development. Yet the process of formulating short- and long-term goals, realizing ambition and coping with disappointments is essentially the same throughout life. The elderly have as much need to adapt to their surroundings as anyone else, but where there is mental or physical deterioration the ability to adjust is diminished.

Activity or disengagement

The recognition that some people have difficulty in adapting as they grow older has prompted considerable discussion on the nature of this change. In the early 1960s the theory was put forward that natural disengagement of society and the individual from each other was not only desirable for successful ageing but was inevitable, and should be regarded as the normal pattern. It was felt to be an essential adjustment that would conserve the elderly person's dwindling physical and mental resources. By contrast the activity, 'engaged' theory holds that most people maintain the same level of activity as they age, that decline of activity reflects ill health and not ageing as such, and that high levels of activity are reflected in a more successful old age (Palmore and Maddox, 1977). Most of the evidence, in particular the Duke longitudinal study, suggests that in Western society the activity theory is more appropriate. Over a 10-year period men showed little or no reduction in activity or life satisfaction, though for women there was a small decline in both activity and satisfaction. Although most people drop certain activities as they grow older they take up new ones instead, so that the overall level for individuals remains fairly constant. Certainly there appears to be a close correlation between a high

11

morale and high levels of activity. However, some elderly people disengage and express considerable life satisfaction. Much depends on their cultural background and previous life styles, so that in India it excites little comment if a man at retirement age withdraws from society, leaves his family and becomes a mendicant.

Loneliness

With increasing age there is a greater chance of death of one's spouse, and at this time there is an increased risk of suicide. Although elderly people who live alone are more likely to complain of loneliness, single people are less likely to be lonely than those who have been widowed, divorced or separated. It would seem that desolation, rather than isolation, is the main feature of loneliness, and it is common to find people in residential homes who complain of loneliness despite the constant presence of other residents. The feeling that there is no friend or relative who cares for them, and a sense of exclusion from the rest of society, are common.

Intelligence

It has become apparent in recent years that there is no simple correlation between advancing years and declining intelligence. Many of the preconceptions are based on Wechsler's cross-sectional study with the Wechsler Adult Intelligence Scale (WAIS), which showed a peak of mental ability in the mid-20s and a steady decline after the age of 30. Cross-sectional work not only produces errors because of the differences between generations caused by variables such as educational standards, length of time at school, standards of housing, nutrition and public health, but also, in the case of the elderly, it does not allow for a decline in physical health. A quasi-longitudinal study has shown no sign of decline; instead IQ scores increased slightly up to the age of 50 and thereafter there was only a very small decline. It is acknowledged that the decline shown in cross-sectional studies may be 'an artifact which merely reflects and catalogues the differences in the sociocultural milieu and experiences of the different generations' (Matarazzo, 1972). However, longitudinal studies are also beset with problems since only the brightest, physically healthiest and most highly motivated subjects remain in the study for any length of time.

It is clear that even mild, asymptomatic illness can reduce performance on the WAIS. Untreated hypertensives do less well than those who are free of disease and whose hypertension is medically controlled. In experiments designed to test the efficacy of pilots at high altitudes whose oxygen supply fails there is, for the more difficult tasks, a direct correlation between reduced cerebral oxygenation and impaired mental performance (Eisdorfer, 1977).

Most longitudinal studies do not show any systematic intellectual decline during old age except for an apparent difficulty in learning. Wechsler suggested that ageing produced a more rapid loss on performance-type tests (digit substitution, picture completion and block design) than on mental skills such as information, vocabulary and comprehension; this indicates that the elderly performed badly on tasks that emphasize speed.

Age and performance

The slowing of performance with age is largely due to slowing of central, decision-making processes rather than in the execution of movements (Welford, 1962). In addition to the role of cardiac insufficiency in prolonging reaction time, there are several other explanations to account for the slowing of decision with age (Welford, 1977).

(1) Reduced signal-to-noise ratio in the brain.
    Reduction in sensory afferents, loss of active brain cells and an increase in spontaneous random neural activity with age ('neural noise') would tend to blur the perception of signals and the making of decisions.
(2) Slowing of EEG rhythms.
    Correlation between reaction time and age can be accounted

13

for by the correlation between alpha-cycle time and age.

(3) Difficulty in manipulating mental data.

Reaction times rise faster with age if, instead of a simple response to a signal, there is an intermediate process such as responding to a signal on the right with a movement of the left hand.

(4) Monitoring of response.

Reaction time to a solitary signal changes relatively little with age but the slowing with age becomes marked when the signals are continuous. This is probably because there is a greater tendency for the elderly to monitor their previous performance before shifting their attention to a new signal.

(5) Caution.

The greater tendency of the elderly to monitor their performance leads to an emphasis on accuracy rather than speed. Indeed they may become more accurate than young subjects.

REFERENCES

Age Concern Research Unit (1977). *Profiles of the Elderly.* Vol. 1, (Mitcham, Surrey: Age Concern)

BASW Working Party (1977). Social work with the elderly. *Social Work Today*, **8**(27), 8

Busse, E. W. (1977). Theories of aging. In E. W. Busse and E. Pffeiffer (eds). *Behaviour and Adaptation in Late Life.* 2nd edn. (Boston: Little, Brown & Co.)

Eisdorfer, C. (1977). Intelligence and cognition in the aged. In E. W. Busse and E. Pfeiffer (eds.). *Behaviour and Adaptation in Late Life.* 2nd edn. (Boston: Little, Brown & Co.)

Hall, D. A. (1976). *The Ageing of Connective Tissue.* (London: Academic Press)

Hayflick, L. (1976). The cell biology of human aging. *N. Engl. J. Med.*, **295**, 1302

Matarazzo, J. D. (1972). *Wechsler's Measurement and Appraisal of Adult Intelligence.* 5th edn. (Baltimore: Williams and Wilkins Co.)

McKeown, T. (1976). *The Role of Medicine*. (London: Rock Carling Fellowship. Nuffield Provincial Hospitals Trust)

Palmore, E. and Maddox, G. L. (1977). Sociological aspects of ageing. In E. W. Busse and E. Pfeiffer (eds.). *Behaviour and Adaptation in Late Life*. 2nd edn. (Boston: Little, Brown & Co.)

Pfeiffer, E. (1977). Sexual behaviour in old age. In E. W. Busse and E. Pfeiffer (eds.). *Behaviour and Adaptation in Late Life*. 2nd edn. (Boston: Little, Brown & Co.)

Welford, A. T. (1962). On changes of performance with age. *Lancet*, **i,** 335

Welford, A. T. (1977). Causes of slowing of performance with age. In I. R. Mackay (ed.). *Interdisciplinary Topics in Gerontology*, **11,** 43. (Basel: Karger)

2
Special features of disease in old age

Two opposing types of change take place concurrently in organs and bodily systems throughout life. In earlier years the changes produced by evolution or growth are the most readily apparent, whereas in later life the changes associated with involution or atrophy of the tissues predominate. Many of the special features of disease in old age are consequences of the structural and functional alterations which occur in the body in senescence.

With advancing years the maintenance and repair of bodily tissues gradually become less affective, with the result that cells die and organ function declines. Bodily systems age differentially and this leads to individual variations in the rate of decline in function in these systems. Such variations in the degree of involution have been called by Sir James Paget 'errors in the chronometry of life'. There are two important consequences of this process: a lack of uniformity in the biological age of different organs and an increasing divergence between one individual and another.

Physiological performance

For the most part the effects of age on organ functions have been investigated on the basis of cross-sectional studies in which physiological performances in individuals of different ages are compared. The findings from these studies must be interpreted with caution, since the age differences which they reveal do not necessarily represent true age-changes affecting all individuals. Longitudinal studies are required, in which measurements made in the same individuals are repeated at intervals of time, in order to interpret the pattern of true age-changes. For obvious reasons few such studies have been undertaken over a prolonged period of time.

TABLE 1

AGE DECREMENTS IN PHYSIOLOGICAL PERFORMANCE

Physiological function	*Percentage reduction at age 80*
Nerve conduction velocity	15
Cardiac output – resting	30
Vital capacity	50
Renal blood flow	50
Maximum breathing capacity	60
Maximum work rate	70
Maximum oxygen uptake	70

Data from Shock and his colleagues, Gerontology Research Centre, Baltimore (see Shock, 1972).

The figures represent the percentage reduction in the mean values at age 80 compared with the mean values of subjects aged 30.

Shock and his colleagues (1972) in Baltimore have carried out measurements of physiological performances both in cross-sectional and longitudinal studies. Some of the results of these investigations are summarized in Table 1. It will be seen from this table that the effects of age vary in different bodily systems. The average decrements range from 15% for nerve conduction velocity to 70% for oxygen

18

uptake during maximum exercise. The greatest age decrements occur in tests carried out when stress is imposed on the organism, particularly in those functions requiring the coordinated activity of a number of systems. Although there is considerable variation in the rate of decline between individuals it is likely that deterioration in function is a universal phenomenon. That this is so has been shown from a few longitudinal studies: for example, Rowe and his colleagues (1976) have investigated renal function by repeated measurements in individuals of different ages, and they have shown a decline in function closely parallel to that revealed by cross-sectional studies. This deterioration in renal excretory power has a direct relevance to drug therapy in old age (see Chapter 16) since plasma levels of drugs for which the main route of elimination from the body is through renal excretion are likely to be elevated when the drug is given in conventional doses appropriate for the normal adult.

Physiological and pathological ageing

Variations in the degree of involution and consequent decline in function may at times be so accentuated as to become pathological and the result is a state which is obviously a departure from normal old age. In the older individual the clinician must attempt to differentiate the physiological changes due to normal ageing from a decrement in function which constitutes a pathological condition. In some instances the distinction is largely academic, but in others it has considerable relevance to the overall management of the patient. A few examples of these difficulties facing the clinician may be mentioned.

In the eye during the fifth decade the ability to change the focal length of the lens becomes impaired as a result of degenerative changes in the muscles of accommodation and of loss in elasticity of the lens. Whereas in a young person the focal length can be changed by 14 or more diopters, in persons over the age of 50 the maximum change may be only 1 diopter. In practice it matters little whether this impairment of accommodation leading to difficulty in near vision (presbyopia) be regarded as physiological or pathological, since the lengthening of the focus of the lens can be corrected by appropriate spectacles. It is of interest, however, that the change in power of accommodation can be used as a measure of the rate of ageing, and it can be included in an ageing test-battery as suggested by Comfort (1969). Moreover, there is some evidence that those individuals who show an accelerated development of presbyopia also show a more rapid rate of ageing in other organs, particularly in the vascular system (Bernstein and Bernstein, 1945).

Both cross-sectional and longitudinal studies show that ageing occurs in the skeleton. After the age of 35 loss of bone tissue in both sexes leads to a diminution in radiographic density of bone and thinning of the cortex of the long bones. This process becomes accelerated in women after the menopause with the result that by the time old age is reached women have lost more bone than have men. This skeletal rarefaction (osteopenia) is of little consequence to the individual unless as a result of a fall he or she sustains a fracture of the femoral neck, or in the case of the spine minor trauma leads to a crush fracture of a vertebral body. As the pathogenesis of osteoporosis becomes better understood and effective treatment becomes available it is clearly important that a distinction should be made between physiological ageing in bone and pathological osteoporosis at a stage before fracture occurs.

Cross-sectional studies show that intellectual function declines with age. Using Raven's Progressive Matrices for the measurement of intellectual performance in different ages the results can be expressed in the form of percentile ranking curves. The maximum performance is at the age of 30 years; thereafter there is a steady decline with the mean performance at 65 years about 25% less than at the age of 30. Furthermore the curves show a divergence with increasing age and the decline in the lower percentiles occurs at a more rapid rate than in the higher percentiles. The interpretation of these findings is difficult, and it must be emphasized that longitudinal studies of intellectual function show that the decline is less rapid than that revealed by cross-sectional studies (see page 12). The neurohistological changes in the brain which accompany ageing include an increase in lipofuscin pigment and the presence of neurofibrillary tangles and senile plaques. These changes are most apparent in the brains of very old people although they are not invariably present. They are, however, always present in the brains of patients dying of senile (Alzheimer-type) dementia. It is probable that there are both qualitative and quantitative differences between normal mental ageing and senile dementia, but the clinician often has difficulty in recognizing the early stages of a dementing process.

The extent to which the rates of physiological decline in function in bodily systems can be altered by favourable or adverse environmental influences is at present unknown. The fact that the downward trend in mental performance with age is greater in the lower percentiles than in the upper has been taken to mean that the decline is more rapid in those with poorer intellectual performance earlier in life and this may be related to lack of use of mental faculties. Some support for this hypothesis is to be found in the work of Heron and Chown (1967) who have studied intellectual function in healthy subjects of different ages in various socioeconomic groups in the population. The findings indicate that there is a differential fall-off with age in non-verbal intelligence with those in the higher occupations showing a slower rate of decline. This matter merits further investigation as it is clearly important to determine whether the continued exercise of mental skills during working life will prevent or slow deterioration. A similar problem exists in relation to muscle strength, which is known to decrease more rapidly in those engaged in sedentary occupations. There is evidence that the maintenance of physical activity, and even increasing it, can slow the rate of decline.

At present we have no precise method for separating that fraction of the decrease in physiological performance which is due to intrinsic processes from that which is due to environmental stresses in earlier life. This is because few of the older people who are examined in cross-sectional studies will have escaped the effects of exposure to disease and accidents. Longitudinal studies will provide the best means of making this distinction and help to identify those environmental influences which have a particularly deleterious effect on the ageing of the individual. A few people, by the good fortune of their genetic inheritance, or perhaps even more by their greater adaptability to internal and external stresses, reach an advanced old age retaining their

21

mental faculties and maintaining well their physical activities. Can what is achieved by these elite become the characteristic of the majority of individuals?

IMPAIRMENT OF HOMEOSTASIS

Under resting conditions the normal old person can maintain constant internal environment within physiological limits which are similar to those found in the young person. Thus blood glucose levels, plasma pH, plasma volume and osmotic pressure are characteristics which under basal conditions show little change with advancing age. Nevertheless, homeostasis of the internal environment is impaired, as shown by a diminished ability to react to stress. The clinical consequences of these age-changes in homeostasis are discussed in later chapters, but a few examples may be mentioned here.

Blood glucose

When a glucose load is imposed in both the oral and intravenous glucose tolerance tests the rise in blood glucose levels is greater and the return to resting levels is slower in older people compared with the young. This pattern in old age is associated with a decreased sensitivity of the pancreatic beta cells to hyperglycaemia and consequent sluggish insulin release (Andres, 1973) and possibly to diminished insulin sensitivity (Soerjodibroto *et al.*, 1979) due to decreased glucoreceptor response to insulin action at the cell membrane. These findings are of direct relevance to the diagnosis of diabetes mellitus in old age (see Chapter 11); if criteria which are used for the diagnosis of diabetes on the results of glucose tolerance tests in younger adults are employed for the elderly a high proportion of the old-age population will have 'chemical' diabetes. The clinician may be reluctant to treat a patient for diabetes on the basis of glucose intolerance shown by the stress of a glucose load, and it has been suggested that there should be an upward revision of standards of normality with age for the 2 h level in the GTT (Royal College of General Practitioners, 1970).

Nevertheless longitudinal studies of glucose tolerance conducted over a period of 10 years show that a significant percentage of patients with an initial GTT abnormality convert to florid diabetes within 10 years, although many remain unchanged and some even become normal (Birmingham Diabetes Survey Working Party, 1976).

Plasma pH

Similar impairments in the rate of recovery of older subjects following displacing stimuli have also been shown in respect of plasma pH, which under basal conditions has a similar value in the old and the young. The oral administration of 10 g of ammonium chloride to a young subject will produce a reduction in the plasma pH of approximately 0.05 in $1\frac{1}{2}$ h with complete recovery to the resting level by the end of 8–10 h. In the 80-year-old, however, the same dose produces a change of about three times this amount and recovery to the resting value takes 24–72 h (Shock, 1972). This impairment of homeostatic capacity makes the elderly more prone to the effects of metabolic acidosis.

Autonomic nervous system

More serious consequences of impairment of homeostatic capacity are seen when the function of the organism as a whole is affected by decline in physiological performance in several bodily systems. Thus an age-related impairment of function in the autonomic nervous system has been demonstrated in both cross-sectional and longitudinal studies (see Chapter 5). Deep body temperature falls with advancing age and hypothermia is more likely to be induced in the old compared with the young on exposure to even mild–moderate cold stress. There are two additional factors which contribute to the greater liability to hypothermia in old age, namely an impaired cold defence due to diminished or absent shivering in response to cold, and impaired thermal perception with consequent decreased awareness of a cold environment.

Impairment of blood pressure regulation in old age is also a

23

consequence of decline of function in the autonomic nervous system. A fall in systolic pressure of 20 mmHg or more has been demonstrated in 14% of the elderly population (Exton-Smith, 1977). By comparison postural hypotension is rare in younger people and when present it is usually associated with such diseases as Wernicke's encephalopathy, diabetic autonomic neuropathy, tabes dorsalis and the Shy–Drager syndrome. Moreover in old age there is often a complex inter-relationship between factors due to deterioration in other systems which account for the serious consequences of postural hypotension. Whereas in young people autoregulation within the cerebral circulation will maintain cerebral blood flow even when systolic pressure decreases by as much as 60 mmHg, in the older person much smaller decreases will produce cerebral ischaemia owing to an impaired capacity of cerebral circulatory autoregulation. In addition, Overstall and his colleagues (1978) have shown that subjects with postural hypotension have an increase in body sway which contributes to the liability to fall, and this is unaffected by the level of blood pressure. Thus in clinical practice important consequences of impaired postural control of blood pressure may be cerebral ischaemia, such manifestations as acute mental confusion, focal neurological disturbances and falls which in turn may lead to hypothermia (if the individual remains on the floor unattended in a cold room) and to fracture, especially in the old person whose bones are brittle due to osteoporosis.

Decline in function and mortality

Thus we have seen that the morphological and functional involution which is a characteristic of ageing affects most of the organs of the body and leads to a gradual decline in the performance of the individual. This decline in function can be viewed as a decreased adaptation between the individual and his environment, and this in turn is reflected in an increased morbidity and mortality. In recent years many attempts have been made (for example, Strehler and Mildvan, 1960) to relate the linear decline in physiological functions to the exponential increase in mortality with age which Gompertz (1825) has shown to occur in humans after middle age.

ALTERED REACTIONS TO DISEASE

Problems in diagnosis arise not only from difficulties in distinguishing physiological and pathological processes, but also from differences in the clinical manifestations of illness in old age.

Confusional states

Mental confusion often dominates the clinical picture. It is a consequence of the lessened tolerance of the ageing brain to the stress brought about by disease in other bodily systems, by altered pharmacodynamic effects of many drugs and by changes in the old person's familiar environment. Hodkinson (1973) in a study of mental impairment in the elderly sponsored by the Royal College of Physicians has shown that important precipitating factors in the development of confusional states are pneumonia, cardiac failure, urinary tract infection, carcinomatosis and hypokalaemia. He also showed that the main predisposing influences are pre-existing dementia, defective hearing and vision, Parkinsonism and advanced age. Thus although confusional states can occur in older people who were previously mentally normal they are much more likely to occur in those whose mental faculties are already impaired by organic brain disease or by disorder of the special senses.

Variation in presentation

There are other modifications in presentation of illness due to different reactions to morbid processes of organs undergoing involution. Thus a few diseases are more acute. For example, appendicitis in the older patient has a fulminating course with the rapid development of gangrene and peritonitis. Atrophy of lymphoid tissue which predisposes to the rapid spread of infection, and the presence of arteriosclerotic mesenteric vessels which readily become occluded by thrombosis, are probably the main factors which lead to this atypical clinical picture.

25

Far more diseases, however, appear to be more benign and undergo slow evolution. For example, in carcinoma of the breast the neoplastic process can be so slow in development that the general condition is well maintained over many years and often the patient ultimately succumbs to some unrelated disorder.

The insidious onset and the 'silent' existence of many diseases make their 'benign' nature more apparent than real. Thus the patient with chronic fibroid phthisis may mention only the non-specific complaint of general weakness; he may have little or no cough, expectoration, fever or night sweats so that the diagnosis is missed until the disease has reached an advanced stage. A benign giant gastric ulcer measuring 5 cm or more in diameter may cause only mild discomfort in the left hypochondrium, and the first indication of its presence may be either perforation or severe haematemesis. Cardiac infarction may have few of the dramatic features such as severe pain and shock seen in middle-aged individuals; in old age it may present with a confusional state, general weakness or a slight increase in breathlessness. The reason for the diminished sensitivity to pain in old age is ill understood, and certain conditions such as cholelithiasis, peritonitis following a perforated viscus and fracture of the femoral neck may be accompanied by so little discomfort that the diagnosis is delayed or missed altogether.

MULTIPLE PATHOLOGICAL PROCESSES

Classical medical teaching, based largely on the experience of illness in younger people, has always stressed the importance of unifying into a single diagnosis all the findings from the history, clinical examination and laboratory investigations. Such an approach is inappropriate in clinical practice in the elderly, the majority of whom suffer from multiple disorders.

System interaction

There are several reasons for multiple pathology in old age and one of the most important has already been discussed; namely, the stress of a disease in one bodily system leading to disorder in another system in which ageing or a pathological process has already produced a deterioration in functional capacity. Cardiac failure is often precipitated by a respiratory infection in an older person whose cardiac reserve is already diminished by coronary disease and myocardial ischaemia. Cardiac infarction and paroxysmal disorders of heart rhythm may lead to changes in the cerebral circulation sufficient to cause mental deterioration or hemiplegia in the absence of thrombosis in a cerebral vessel. Prolonged hypoglycaemia, especially when induced by long-acting anti-diabetic agents such as chlorpropamide, may produce mental and neurological disturbances which simulate those due to acute cerebrovascular disease.

Co-existent degenerative disorders

Multiple pathological processes also occur in the elderly on account of the coincidence of degenerative disorders and on account of the accumulation of injuries. Obesity, hypertension, arteriosclerosis, diabetes mellitus, diverticulosis, spondylosis and osteoarthritis are common conditions which may occur simultaneously in one individual. On such a background of degeneration affecting several systems, acute illness such as cardiac infarction or stroke may develop at any time and necessitate admission of the patient to hospital. Cancer, myxoedema and pernicious anaemia become more frequent with increasing age and are probably due to an age-related decline in the immune system. Osteomalacia and other manifestations of small intestinal malabsorption sometimes develop many years after partial gastrectomy for duodenal ulcer.

UNREPORTED ILLNESS

Sheldon (1948) was one of the first physicians to carry out a comprehensive survey of the elderly at home. In a random sample

27

of the population of women over the age of 60 and men over the age of 65 a high incidence of disabilities was found; 2% were bedridden, 8% had disabilities which confined them to the house and just over one-fifth had only limited outside movement. Rheumatism affected 55% and painful conditions of the feet were present in 40%. Vertigo, liability to fall and difficulty in getting about in the dark were especially common in very elderly women and were experienced by 70% of female subjects over the age of 85. About 5% of the old people had sustained a stroke, and some mental abnormality was present in nearly 20%. Similar findings were reported by Hobson and Pemberton (1955) whose study of the elderly population in Sheffield included a dietary assessment and biochemical investigations as well as a full medical examination. Williamson and his colleagues (1964) carried out a full physical and psychiatric examination of elderly men and women on the lists of three general practices in Scotland, with the aim of ascertaining to what extent the health and social needs of old people were being met. They found that men had a mean of 3.26 disabilities of which 1.87 were not known to the general practitioner, and women a mean of 3.42 disabilities of which 2.03 were not known (see Figure 1).

Dementia, depression, locomotor disorders, urinary tract diseases, anaemia, failing vision and deafness were particularly common and unreported. The findings of this study indicate that the unmet need for general practitioner care is high, and the main reason for this is that old people do not report their disabilities until they are advanced. Thus a general practitioner service based on the self-reporting of illness is severely handicapped in meeting the needs of old people. But Williamson emphasizes the importance of the early detection of disease because preventive medicine is at least as important in old age as it is in earlier life, and there are few conditions which medical and social measures applied soon enough will not help.

Cartwright (1967) has also examined the extent to which old people fail to seek advice when suffering from chronic conditions. A high proportion of the subjects had painful disability of the feet, defects of eyesight and hearing and backache, all lasting for more than 3 months. Yet as many as 46% of those with backache had not consulted anyone about the complaint. She also found that old people living alone received the least amount of medical attention, and 40% had not seen their general practitioners during the previous 12 months; whereas for those who lived with people of a younger generation, 47% had consulted their doctor five or more times during the year.

Preventive medicine forms an important aspect of the practice of geriatrics. Facilities for early diagnosis and for adequate treatment are required to prevent or to delay progress of a disorder, to reduce the chance of development of 'vicious circles of regressive change' in which a lesion in one bodily system leads to disorder in another, and, most important, to institute appropriate medical or social measures to prevent the occurrence of dependency.

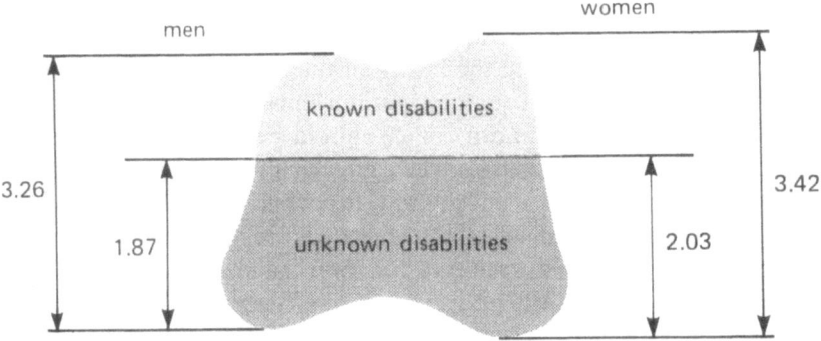

Figure 1 Unreported illness in the elderly population (after Williamson *et al.*, 1964)

THE AIMS OF TREATMENT

For many of the diseases which afflict the elderly complete 'cure' is rarely possible. Yet a more thorough investigation of the elderly patient reveals that much disability which might otherwise be attributed to senility is due to specific disease processes, and these may be capable of mitigation by appropriate treatment. There are also many

29

conditions which in themselves are not directly lethal, but they can lead if neglected to progressive disablement. Take for example an elderly woman who suffers from obesity, the residual effects of a stroke, painful disabilities of the feet, anaemia, oesophageal hiatus hernia and diverticular disease. Effective management depends upon the recognition of the distinction between disability and the diseases which cause it and the assessment of the disability, both physical and mental, on a functional basis.

Disease and disability

When a full clinical assessment of all the underlying pathological processes has been made by medical examination, supported by the appropriate investigations, treatment should be aimed first at the more serious conditions affecting the health of the patient. The therapeutic regimen should consist of the minimum number of the most effective drugs (see Chapter 16) and a choice should be made of those drugs which are least likely to cause adverse effects. The management of disability and the restoration of optimum function are the concern of the rehabilitation team, and some of the methods are described in Chapter 15. Even the partial restoration of function may make a considerable difference between a useful and a useless life. It is particularly relevant to geriatric practice that disease in its broadest sense should be regarded as a maladjustment between an individual and his environment. Social relationships and domestic conditions are so inextricably linked with the medical aspects of the patient's illness that return home from hospital and satisfactory domestic resettlement can only be achieved when adverse social and physical factors in the home environment have been corrected. The general practitioner must retain the central role in caring for the patient at home, and successful management depends upon the fullest collaboration at all stages in the patient's illness between the hospital geriatric team and the primary care team. Many patients can benefit from attendance at the Geriatric Day Hospital (Brocklehurst, 1970): the duration of in-patient treatment can be shortened and treatment by the rehabilitation team can

30

be continued. In other cases maximal functional capacity, which has been attained only after months of treatment, can be maintained.

The elderly in hospital

The need for hospital admission for the severely ill elderly patient is not usually in dispute, and there are many other patients with less serious illnesses for whom admission is necessary because satisfactory treatment at home is precluded by adverse social circumstances. For the severely ill old person, who is in fact in almost every way totally dependent upon others, the change in environment brought about by admission to hospital is usually to the patient's ultimate good. Emergency and complicated treatment can be effectively carried out. It is obvious, however, that when the acute phase of the illness has passed the rigid system of traditional hospital care is not well suited to the patient's full rehabilitation. For this the encouragement of initiative, the provision of opportunities for independent action, and the attainment of self-reliance are all important. Moreover, the patient with a long-term disability and the elderly infirm tend to suffer a decline in their functional capabilities and their self-sufficiency in the ordinary hospital ward. Modifications of patterns of hospital care have been developed into systems of progressive patient care for the elderly (Exton-Smith, 1962). These schemes have been adopted by the majority of geriatric departments with consequent improvement in efficiency and benefit to older patients.

Rest and activity

The correct approach to the problem of hospital treatment of the elderly must be based on a consideration of the desirability of rest. In a general ward it is usually taken for granted that the younger hospital patients should be in bed, but unnecessary immobilization in the case of the elderly is frequently disastrous and may end in permanent bedfastness.

Ill-advised and prolonged immobilization of elderly patients may have the following harmful effects:

31

(a) Psychological

As a result of boredom and mental apathy the patient neglects his personal toilet and loses all self-respect. With further deterioration incontinence usually develops and adds to the degradation. Lack of mental stimulation, especially in those with impairment of vision and hearing, leads to a form of sensory deprivation. The final stage is a complete disintegration of the personality, which is all the more regrettable because it cannot be reversed.

(b) Physical

The joints become stiff and contractures develop, particularly in the hamstrings, causing fixed flexion of the knees, and in the calf muscles producing foot-drop. Pressure sores develop in the skin at sites over bony prominences. Constipation due to inactivity and unawareness of rectal distension lead to faecal impaction. With the increased liability to infection, hypostatic pneumonia and pyelocystitis may occur. Prolonged immobilization also favours the development of osteoporosis and deep vein thrombosis.

In order to minimize these hazards the period during which an elderly patient is confined to bed must be reduced as far as possible. Many of the accepted reasons for keeping patients in bed are not valid for the elderly. Thus early ambulation, now widely accepted following surgery, is of benefit in a variety of medical conditions including hemiplegia, Parkinsonism, arthritis, spondylosis, osteoporosis, varicose ulcers and in certain respiratory and cardiac disorders. Although the practice of early mobilization of patients with physical disabilities initially imposes a heavier strain on the nursing and remedial staff, once increased activity is established the patient can take responsibility for his personal hygeine and so later the work of the nurses and remedial therapists is lightened.

Value of hospital treatment

Arnold and Exton-Smith (1962) have clearly demonstrated the value of hospital treatment when the results are assessed in terms of functional capacity. In their study of 212 patients (whose mean age was nearly 80 years) discharged from a geriatric department 60% were improved by treatment and most of these were found to have maintained their improvement when assessed 3 months later. These results are comparable with those reported in a study carried out in four Scottish hospital of patients of all ages (of whom only 18% were over the age of 65); 88% showed clinical improvement or cure in hospital, but after 3 months only 55% maintained their improvement. The encouraging results in the geriatric series can be attributed to the careful planning of the therapeutic and rehabilitation programmes for the individual patient and a close collaboration between the hospital geriatric and community health services.

REFERENCES

Andres, R. (1973). Ageing and carbohydrate metabolism. In L. A. Carlson (ed.). *Nutrition and Old Age.* (Stockholm: Almquist and Wiksell)

Arnold, J. and Exton-Smith, A. N. (1962). The geriatric department and community: value of hospital treatment in the elderly. *Lancet*, **ii**, 551

Bernstein, F. and Bernstein, M. (1945). Law of physiologic ageing as derived from long range data on refraction of the human eye. *Arch. Ophthalmol.*, **34**, 378

Birmingham Diabetes Survey Working Party (1976). Ten-year follow up report on Birmingham diabetes survey of 1961

Brocklehurst, J. C. (1970). *The Geriatric Day Hospital.* (London: King Edward's Hospital Fund)

Cartwright, A. (1967). *Patients and their Doctors.* (London: Routledge & Kegan Paul)

Comfort, A. (1969). A test battery to measure ageing-rate in man. *Lancet*, **ii**, 1411

Exton-Smith, A. N. (1962). Progressive patient care in geriatrics. *Lancet*, **i**, 260

Exton-Smith, A. N. (1977). Functional consequences of ageing: clinical manifestations. In A. N. Exton-Smith and J. Grimley Evans (eds.). *Care of the Elderly: Meeting the Challenge of Dependency* (London: Academic Press)

Gompertz, B. (1825). On the nature of the function expressive of the law of human mortality and on a new model of determining life contingencies.

Phil. Trans. R. Soc. Lond. (Biol.), **115,** 513

Heron, A. and Chown, S. (1967). *Age and Function.* (London: Churchill)

Hobson, W. and Pemberton, J. (1955). *Health of the Elderly at Home.* (London: Butterworth)

Hodkinson, H. M. (1973). Mental impairment in the elderly. *J. Roy. Coll. Phys., Lond.,* **7,** 305

Overstall, P. W., Johnson, A. L. and Exton-Smith, A. N. (1978). Instability and falls in the elderly. *Age and Ageing,* **7,** Suppl. 92

Rowe, J. W., Andres, R., Tobin, J. D., Norris, A. H. and Shock, N. W. (1976). The effect of age on creatinine clearance in men: a cross-sectional and longitudinal study. *J. Gerontol.,* **31,** 155

Royal College of General Practitioners (1970). Five year follow-up report on the Birmingham diabetes survey of 1962. *Br. Med. J.,* **3,** 301

Sheldon, J. H. (1948). *The Social Medicine of Old Age.* (London: Oxford University Press)

Shock, N. W. (1972). Energy metabolism, caloric intake and physical activity of the ageing. In L. A. Carlson (ed.). *Nutrition in Old Age.* (Stockholm: Almquist & Wicksell)

Soerjodibroto, W. S., Hearn, C. R. . and Exton-Smith, A. N. (1979). Glucose tolerance, plasma insulin levels and insulin sensitivity in elderly patients. *Age and Ageing,* **8,** 65

Strehler, B. L. and Mildvan, A. S. (1960). General theory of mortality and ageing. *Science,* **132,** 14

Williamson, J., Stokoe, I. H., Gray, S., Fisher, M., Smith, A., Mcghee, A. and Stephenson, E. (1964). Old people at home – their unreported needs. *Lancet,* **i,** 1117

3
Mental disorders

There is usually some atrophy of the brain, particularly the frontal lobes, with shrinkage of the gyri and widening of sulci. Micro-scopically there is an accumulation in neurones of *lipofuscin*, a yellow-brown pigment that although probably not harmful in itself, indicates a reduction in efficiency of the nerve cell's metabolism. It is increased in the presence of degenerative disease.

Neuronal fallout

It has been claimed that at the age of 30 the human brain contains 20 billion cells and that this number decreases by 0.8% a year. However, there is much controversy on the subject and although it is probable that some cells are lost from certain areas, such as the cerebellum, there is little evidence of a widespread loss. In some ways this is sur-prising, since neurones are incapable of dividing and any loss during life cannot be made good. What is more important in normal ageing is not the loss of neurones but the decline in the quality of the nerve cell processes, and this probably reflects deteriorating homeostatic stab-ility (Bowen and Davison, 1978).

Blood supply

Although cortical atrophy is accelerated by ischaemia there is no evidence that atherosclerotic vascular disease is the cause of ageing changes in the brain. Cerebral oxygen consumption is the same in young subjects as it is in non-arteriosclerotic elderly subjects. It is the functional activity of the neurone that determines blood supply (Bowen and Davison, 1978).

Lewy bodies

These are spheres of hyaline within neurones. They are present mainly in the pigmented neurones of the basal ganglia and their numbers are considerably increased in idiopathic Parkinson's disease.

Senile plaques

These begin as groups of degenerating neurites, mature, become denser and accumulate amyloid.

Neurofibrillary tangles

These are argyrophilic bundles of fibrillary material that appear within the cytoplasm of neurones, particularly in the hippocampus.

Granulovacuolar degeneration

This is, as its name indicates, a small intracytoplasmic vacuole with a central dense granule. It is found only in neurones and most commonly affects pyramidal cells in the hippocampus.

Senile plaques, neurofibrillary tangles and granulovacuolar degeneration are commonly found, in descending order of frequency, in the brains of normal people over the age of 65 years. They represent different degenerative changes and are not related to each other either in their frequency or in their distribution. This triad of changes is also

36

characteristically found before the age of 35 in the brains of patients with Down's syndrome; also in Alzheimer's disease and senile dementia. The difference between the pathology of normal ageing and dementia is mainly quantitative; the triad of changes being more numerous and widespread in dementia.

DEMENTIA

This may be defined as a global loss of intellectual function that is usually irreversible. It affects approximately one in ten people over the age of 65 (half of them severely) and one in five over the age of 80 (Kay, Beamish and Roth, 1964). The sex incidence is approximately equal, though more women are affected because more survive into old age.

TABLE 1
CLASSIFICATION OF DEMENTIA (Chronic brain failure)

Pre-senile (<60 years)	Alzheimer's
	Pick's
	Huntingdon's chorea
	Jakob – Creutzfeldt
Senile (>60 years)	Senile (primary neuronal, Alzheimer's)
	Multi-infarct (atherosclerotic)
	Mixed senile and multi-infarct
	Miscellaneous – B_{12} and folate deficiency, syphilis, hypo-hyperthyroidism, hypo-, hypercalcaemia, low-pressure hydrocephalus, etc.

Senile dementia

This is the typical, insidious onset, slowly progressive dementia of old age and accounts for about 50% of cases. A further 20% have a combination of changes typical of senile and multi-infarct dementia. The brain is characterized by thinning of the cortical ribbon, which reflects neuronal loss, and a proliferation of senile plaques, neurofibrillary tangles and granulovacuolar degeneration. By measuring biochemical constituents it has been estimated that there is a loss of approximately half the total nerve-cell population, compared with age-matched controls, (Spillane *et al.*, 1977). This contrasts with the negligible neurone loss in normal ageing.

The argument as to whether senile dementia is a distinct disease or an exaggeration of normal ageing continues. The aetiology is unknown and is certainly unconnected with the misleading idea of atherosclerotic vessels gradually strangling the blood supply to the brain. Recently there have been several reports showing that a biochemical abnormality underlies senile dementia. It appears that there is a selective depletion of choline acetyl transferase activity in the cerebral presynaptic cholinergic system. There is also evidence that in normal people the age-related memory loss is due to involvement of central cholinergic pathways (White *et al.*, 1977). The implication is that rational treatment of dementia with centrally acting cholinergic drugs may be possible.

Clinical features
The patient is rarely seen in the early stages, which usually means undiagnosed cases in the community. One survey estimated that 80% of old people with moderate to severe dementia were not known to be demented by their general practitioner. There is no neat division between an old person who is merely forgetful and one who is developing dementia. Many cases of mild memory loss are not so benign as was once thought, and are associated with decreased life expectancy and sometimes progression to dementia. In practice the determining factor is the quality of life and the ability to cope at home. An old lady may not remember the name of the street or the number where she lives, but if she is able to get out to do her shopping, collect her pension and find her way home again, her memory impairment is not yet critical.

Memory The essential problem is a loss of short-term memory, with relative preservation in the early stages of memory for distant events.

38

The patient may forget where he is, the time and even who he is. Consequently he becomes confused and anxious. He may be restless and forever wandering off to look for something, only to get lost and be returned home by neighbours or the police. Neighbours may complain that he knocks on the door in the middle of the night shouting that it is time to get up for work. Delusions that he has been robbed are common, because he puts down his wallet or keys and then cannot remember where he has put them.

Intellect There is increasing difficulty in handling abstract ideas. New ideas are not grasped and there is an inability to learn from experience. Impairment of constructional ability (drawing or building two- or three-dimensional designs) occurs early, but is rarely complained of unless the patient is an artist or architect.

Personality In the early stages there is often an exaggeration of the patient's previous personality traits. Thus he may be more cantankerous and irritable than before or appear to be all sweetness and light, constantly reassuring everyone that everything is all right and that he is perfectly happy.

Antisocial, uninhibited behaviour may cause considerable difficulties for the relatives: the patient defaecating on the carpet, masturbating openly or wandering naked in the street. Depression, as part of the dementia, is quite common, often with bizarre delusions and fluctuating mood.

As the disease progresses the emotions become increasingly shallow and the patient sinks into a profound apathy. Speech becomes meaningless and then dries up altogether. Worsening incontinence and immobility are the rule.

Life expectancy It has been said that life expectancy, for patients who are so dependent that admission to hospital becomes necessary, is 2 years. Death is due to progressive emaciation (despite a good appetite), pressure sores or bronchopneumonia. With skilled nursing, however, it is not unusual for patients to survive twice that time.

Diagnosis

A history of insidious onset of intellectual decline with steady progression and personality deterioration is most important. Great care, though, must be taken not to let 'dementia' become a blanket diagnostic term for all confused elderly people (Roth and Myers, 1969).

TABLE 2
DIFFERENTIAL DIAGNOSES OF DEMENTIA

	Similarities	*Differences*
Depression	apathy; unresponsiveness; memory loss; self neglect; incontinence of urine	often recent and acute onset; memory loss patchy and fluctuates day to day; say 'I don't know' in response to questions; show distress; family and previous history; response to treatment
Toxic confusional states	confusion; disorientation; self-neglect; incontinence of urine	recent, acute onset; clouding of consciousness; drowsiness fluctuates; lucid periods; hallucinations
Paraphrenia	impairment of thinking; apathy; emotional flattening; delusions	memory and intellect intact, hallucinations; primary delusions; feeling of passivity
Dysphasia (tumour or stroke)	talks nonsense; appears confused	rapid onset; focal neurological signs; clouding of consciousness; focal fits

Mental assessment

It is always necessary to make a formal assessment of a patient's mental status and to record it in the notes. Allowance must be made for the patient's level of schooling and poor concentration (Strub and Black, 1977).

Memory

(1) Immediate recall. Test by asking the patient to repeat a number of digits. Start with three and work up. A normal person

should be able to repeat at least seven digits. This also tests the patient's concentration.

(2) Long-term memory. Ask date of First World War, name of monarch, where patient worked, name of spouse.

(3) New learning ability. Give patient a name and address and ask for it to be repeated after 2 minutes (e.g. John Green, 42 West Street).

Orientation   Ask patient his name, age and date of birth; his address, where he is now; time, day, month and year.

Constructional ability   Ask patient to draw a clock, a house and a man. Copy simple shapes. This ability is usually lost early in the course of dementia.

The patient should not be hurried, and it is best to avoid giving the impression that you are asking the questions because you think he is mad. Beginning an interview with the question 'What is the name of the Prime Minister?' may cause the patient some alarm.

Physical examination
In the early stages this is often unremarkable. Note should be made of the patient's general appearance, state of hair, clothes, finger- and toe-nails and whether or not he is incontinent. As the disease progresses bruising and other injuries, due to frequent falls, may be seen. Muscle tone is generally increased and the patient may resist passive movements or cling onto the nurse when turned in bed. The gait is short-stepped and shuffling, or may resemble the apraxic gait described by Petren. Here the patient's feet appear rooted to the ground despite an attempt to walk, and when finally he does walk the steps are short. It is usually possible to get the patient to walk normally by asking him to step over lines drawn at 18-inch intervals on the floor or by going up-stairs. A tendency to lean backwards, due to frontal lobe disease, is often found.

Many primitive reflexes reappear, such as the pout reflex (lips pout when lightly tapped), rooting reflex (head turns towards stimulated side when cheek stroked) and the palmo-mental reflex (a firm scratch along the palm produces a contraction of the ipsilateral mentis muscle in the chin). The glabellar tap is usually positive.

Investigations
The diagnosis of senile dementia is one of exclusion and one must consider the possibility of other rare (but potentially treatable) causes of dementia (see Tables 1 and 2), as well as conditions that may aggravate the patient's confusion.

(1) Full blood count and film.
(2) Serum B_{12} and red cell folate levels.
(3) Urea and creatinine.
(4) Syphilis serology.
(5) Thyroid function tests.
(6) Calcium, inorganic phosphate and alkaline phosphatase.
(7) Chest X-ray.
(8) Brain scan or computerized axial tomography.

Management
Six out of seven demented patients live at home, and apart from the fact that there are not enough institutional beds to admit them all, it is generally in the patient's best interest for him to remain in his own familiar surroundings for as long as possible. One should therefore try to identify these patients early in the course of their disease so that relatives can be consulted and supported.

Demented patients who are ignored do not go away. Instead they present as a crisis (often at weekends) when relatives have reached the end of their tether and are ready to abrogate responsibility for the patient. Removing the patient from his own environment is likely to aggravate his confusion, but the pressure from relatives for some relief may be so strong that there is no practical alternative. On such occasions it should be made clear that the admission is only a temporary one and that the patient will be returning home in a couple of weeks, with additional support from community services.

Paradoxically, if a demented patient abruptly worsens (due to, say, an infection) it is better to admit him promptly for treatment rather than let him deteriorate at home.

Wandering nocturnal disturbance   The a m is to provide the patient with a sufficiently interesting occupation so that he will be tired and ready for sleep at night. This usually means a day centre or day hospital where the activities can be supervised and there is stimulus from other people.

Persistent insomnia may require chlormethiazole 500 mg–1 g nocte or if there is considerable agitation a phenothiazine (e.g. thioridazine 50–75 mg nocte). Too much sedation produces a drowsy, uncooperative patient the next morning, and finding the correct dose is a matter of trial and error. Where there is persistent agitation it is best (before automatically increasing the level of sedation) to review the patient and his treatment so as to ensure that the agitation is not due to irritation from, say, impacted faeces or a distended bladder. Drugs, too, should occasionally be withdrawn to see if they are still effective.

Support for relatives   It is essential that the prime supporter of the patient, whoever he or she is, should feel that their efforts are appreciated and understood, and that practical help is at hand. This may mean daytime relief at day centre or day hospital, domiciliary support from a home help, the incontinent laundry service and occasional hospital admissions to give the supporters a holiday.

Institutional care   Where there is no behavioural disturbance a residential home is the most appropriate place for care. Local authorities differ in their approach to the problem. Some have elderly mentally infirm (EMI) homes, whilst others prefer to mix the residents. There are good arguments on both sides but it is often so distressing for mentally normal old people to have to live with demented residents that some segregation is probably necessary. This does not mean, of course, that mistakes of the past have to be repeated and EMI homes turned into a dumping ground for all the difficult people that no-one else wants. If linked to a geriatric or psychiatric unit and given adequate staffing and medical back-up they have been shown to work well.

Geriatrics

The severely demented patient with behavioural disturbances will usually be admitted to a psychiatric hospital, whilst those who are confined to bed and in need of general nursing care go to the geriatricians. There has been much recent interest in the quality of this continuing care. With the help of relatives, volunteers and professional staff the lives of the patients can be considerably improved by outings, films, reality orientation (Holden and Sinebruchow, 1978) and art therapy. The crucial point is that if the ward has become the patient's home then it should be homely and not run on rigid hospital lines.

Drug treatment of dementia

It has already been mentioned that there is little or no reduction in cerebral blood flow with normal ageing. Blood flow is also unaltered in senile dementia and it is only in multi-infarct dementia that there is a demonstrable reduction in flow rate that is related to the degree of dementia (Hachinski et al., 1975). Thus the use of cerebral vasodilators is only likely to be effective in multi-infarct dementia.

There are many vasoactive drugs available such as alpha-adrenergic blockers, (e.g. dihydro-ergot alkaloids – Hydergine), beta-adrenergic stimulants (e.g. isoxsuprine – Duvadilan), drugs acting directly on vascular smooth muscle (e.g. cyclandelate – Cyclospasmol) and those with combined effects (e.g. naftidrofuryl – Praxilene). Some of these drugs are claimed to be more than vasodilators. Hydergine is said to improve ganglion cell metabolism and normalize disturbed astrocyte metabolism, and Praxilene is believed to elevate ATP levels in the brain (Hyams, 1978). Critical examination of published drug trials, however, shows that none of these drugs does much more than produce very minor symptomatic improvements. Tests of intellect or memory are unchanged.

The one ray of light in this otherwise gloomy therapeutic scene is the recent discovery that a deficit of the cholinergic neurotransmitter underlies the memory defect of senile dementia. In 1974 it was noted by Drachman and Leavitt that the anticholinergic drug scopolamine temporarily produced in young healthy volunteers the same sort of memory defect that characterizes Alzheimer's disease. Attention

44

turned to cholinergic and anticholinesterase drugs, and it was shown in rats that by increasing the amount of choline in the diet there was a corresponding rise of acetylcholine in the brain. Memory in young normal volunteers has been reported to improve temporarily with choline (Sitaram, Weingarten and Gillin, 1978) and physostigmine (Davis *et al.*, 1978).

The trials so far reported on the use of choline in patients with senile dementia have been disappointing, but there is a suggestion of improvement in patients whose disease is still at an early stage (Signoret, Whiteley and Lhermitte, 1978). Work continues with both choline and lecithin (a natural source of choline).

Multi-infarct dementia

This accounts for about 20% of elderly dementia cases and a further 20% where it co-exists with senile dementia. It is more common in men and tends to occur at an earlier age than senile dementia. It is caused by multiple small or large infarcts occurring over many months or years, and is often associated with hypertension (*état lacunaire*) (Hachinski, Lassen and Marshall, 1974).

Clinical
The onset is usually abrupt with an episode of clouding of consciousness associated with the cerebral infarct. Over a few days the patient recovers to a considerable degree, although usually he is left with some impairment. He may then continue like this for weeks or months until there is another acute episode. Thus the patient's decline is step-like, rather than smoothly progressive. The personality is often fairly well preserved and the patient may be unhappily aware of his mental deterioration. Emotional incontinence, with the patient crying or laughing inappropriately, is common.

Physical examination
During the course of the disease focal signs appear: weakness, slowness, marche à petits pas gait, brisk reflexes, extensor plantar responses, pseudo-bulbar signs (dysarthria, dysphagia, weakness of

tongue and palate), apraxia and agnosia.

The patient should be regarded as having transient ischaemic attacks and a search made for hypertension, cardiac dysrhythmias, valvular heart disease and carotid bruits.

Investigations
These are directed towards finding a cause for the recurrent cerebral infarcts and will include an ECG and possibly 24-hour cardiac monitoring (see Chapter 6). Carotid angiograms (which have an appreciable morbidity and mortality) should only be done if the patient is considered fit enough for endarterectomy. Other investigations are the same as for senile dementia.

Treatment
Blood pressure above 160/95 should be gently lowered with diuretics and a beta-blocker. Cardiac dysrhythmias need treating, if necessary with a pacemaker, and the use of anticoagulants considered, if emboli are thought to be the cause of the infarcts. Anticoagulants are clearly dangerous in the hands of a demented patient and there is evidence that aspirin may be a useful alternative.

Miscellaneous causes of dementia

Almost certainly these account for only a small percentage of patients.

Thyroid disease
Both myxoedema and hyperthyroidism can cause dementia, and it should be remembered that classical signs of thyroid disorder are uncommon in the elderly (see Chapter 11).

Vitamin B_{12} or folate deficiency
Dementia has been described in both conditions in the absence of anaemia and neurological signs (see Chapter 12). Borderline low levels of both vitamin B_{12} and folate are not unusual in the elderly, and although they should be treated, hopes of improving a concomitant dementia should not be raised too high.

Syphilis
General paralysis of the insane is rare but the cost of missing it is high. If syphilis serology is positive then the test must be repeated on the cerebrospinal fluid.

Low-pressure (communicating) hydrocephalus
In this rare, but curious, condition the pressure in the cerebrospinal fluid is normal but there is defective resorption of fluid and symmetrical enlargement of the lateral ventricles. It may be idiopathic or secondary to previous subarachnoid haemorrhage, meningitis or head injury.

Characterisically the patient has dementia, gait apraxia and incontinence, but before this triad develops there may be (a) non-specific complaints such as headaches, depression and loss of memory; (b) a tonic foot response of the sole and grasp reflex cf the foot in the absence of a hand reflex; and (c) falls indistinguishable from drop attacks (Botez *et al.*, 1977).

Tumours
These can cause dementia when they damage the cerebral hemispheres. A slowly growing meningioma can closely mimic senile dementia with its insidious onset and gradual progress. Papilloedema is a late sign, and suspicions should be aroused if there is clouding of consciousness, fits or focal neurological signs.

Steel–Richardson–Olszewski syndrome (Progressive supranuclear palsy)
Characteristically the dementia is mild and because of the accompanying extrapyramidal signs the patients are sometimes mis-diagnosed as having Parkinson's disease. Usually there is insidious development of symptoms which include frequent falls; difficulty in walking; dystonic rigidity of face, neck and upper trunk; supranuclear ophthalmoplegia mainly affecting vertical gaze and pseudobulbar signs (Dalziel and Griffiths, 1977).

Dementia has been described in alcoholism, hyper- and hypo-calcaemia, following chronic brain injury (particularly in boxers) and in vitamin B_1 and B_6 deficiencies. Chronic subdural haematoma is discussed on page 50).

Presenile dementia

This is a dementia occurring before the age of 60, but the patient may survive beyond that age.

Alzheimer's disease

Traditionally, this is the name given to the commonest dementia of middle age, whilst the same disease occurring in later life is called senile dementia. The pathology and clinical features are identical.

Pick's disease

This is very rare and is characterized by well-defined areas of cerebral atrophy that are clearly picked out from the remaining areas of normal brain. The main regions involved are the frontal and temporal lobes and often the basal ganglia. There are no useful clinical points to distinguish it from Alzheimer's disease.

Huntington's chorea

There is usually a family history since it is inherited as a simple Mendelian dominant trait, but sporadic cases are not uncommon. Characteristically the onset of dementia and irregular, jerky involuntary movements occurs in the fourth or fifth decade with slow progression towards total motor and mental disability.

The brain is generally atrophied, particularly the caudate nucleus and to a lesser extent the putamen, globus pallidus and frontal lobes. Deficiencies in cerebral tissue of gamma-aminobutyric acid (GABA), its synthesizing enzyme, glutamic acid decarboxylase, and choline acetyl transferase have been shown. Drugs that reduce the activity of dopamine (such as haloperidol, phenothiazines, tetrabenazine and pimozide) may improve the chorea. L-dopa makes it worse.

Jakob–Creutzfeldt disease

This rare cause of dementia typically begins in middle age and runs from a few months to not more than 2 years. Clinically there is a wide variety of neurological abnormalities which include motor and cerebellar signs, myoclonus, spasticity and choreoathetosis. The pathological features are also varied but usually show nerve cell loss, astrocytic proliferation and a spongy state throughout the cerebral cortex. The disease has been transmitted to chimpanzees and (inadvertently) to man. The agent has not been identified but is assumed to be a slow virus.

Vigorous investigation of the younger patient with dementia is worthwhile. One specialist centre found that 15% of patients referred with a diagnosis of presenile dementia had conditions amenable to treatment (Marsden and Harrison, 1972).

TOXIC CONFUSIONAL STATES

Confusion in an old person is similar to fever in a child: it is merely an indicator of illness and not a diagnosis in itself. There is a sudden onset of confusion, falls or incontinence and often no obvious pointer to the underlying condition.

Although the confusion, at first, may mimic dementia there are fluctuations, so that at times the patient is lucid, intellect is intact and memory for the period prior to the illness is clear (see Table 2). Clouding of consciousness, sleepiness and hallucinations can occur. The condition is reversible and the prognosis is therefore good.

Environment
A sudden change in the patient's surroundings, such as a move to a Residential Home, may be a precipitating factor.

Infections
These are common causes and include bronchopneumonia, urinary tract infections and septicaemia.

Cardiovascular
'Silent' myocardial infarction, heart failure and dysrhythmias must be looked for.

Drugs

A major problem in the elderly is their liability to drug toxicity (see Chapter 16). It is usually necessary to question relatives or search the patient's belongings to discover exactly which drugs have been taken. Any recently prescribed drug must be regarded with suspicion.

Alcohol and barbiturates are notorious, but a wide range of drugs including digoxin, antidepressants, tranquillizers and anti-Parkinsonian agents can be responsible.

Metabolic

Dehydration, electrolyte disturbances following surgery, renal or liver failure, hyper- or hypoglycaemia, thyroid disorders and avitaminosis (particularly thiamine deficiency) have all been described as causing toxic confusional states.

Injury

Fractures may be overlooked since the patient will not necessarily complain of pain.

Subdural haematoma is sometimes missed because of failure to consider the possibility. The interval between trauma and admission to hospital can vary from 24 h to 6 months, and unless one is fortunate enough to get a clear account of injury the most useful points from the history are a disturbance of conscious level and headaches. Focal neurological signs (usually a mild hemiparesis) are present at some time in about 80% of patients.

Where there is a strong suspicion of a subdural haematoma it is best to call in a neurosurgeon at an early stage. However the picture is usually not clear-cut and in such cases one should obtain a skull X-ray (simple and worthwhile, but the diagnostic yield is low) an echoencephalogram (simple, but negative results do not exclude the diagnosis since 30% of subdural haematomas are bilateral and thus will not show a shift) and a brain scan (again, false negatives occur). Short of exploratory burr holes, computerized axial tomography is the most reliable diagnostic method (Dronefield, Mead and Langman, 1977).

Management

Treatment is directed at the underlying condition. The patient is nursed in bright surroundings and should not be moved about but allowed to familiarize himself with one part of the ward. If possible a relative or friend should sit with the patient, but otherwise staff must constantly visit and help to reorientate him by explaining what has happened and where he is. It is probably best if all drugs are temporarily withheld until a diagnosis is made.

DEPRESSION

The term depression includes a variety of emotional reactions which range from grief in response to bereavement to endogenous or psychotic depression. It cannot be too strongly emphasized that anxiety and depression themselves, and the symptoms derived from them, are very unpleasant and cause considerable suffering (Post, 1965).

Community surveys show that moderate to severe depression occurs in approximately 15% of the elderly population. Suicide is a serious hazard and several studies reveal that there is a disproportionately high suicide rate amongst the elderly. While the 65-and-over age group represent 10–15% of the general population in most Western societies, they comprise at least 38% of all known suicides.

Clinical manifestations

There is a diversity of clinical symptomatology in depression, and some of the features are shown in Table 3. Not all these features are to be seen in the individual patient, and in old age there tends to be a greater variation between individuals. Attempts have been made to describe the clinical picture under a number of descriptive headings such as: organic depressions, depressive pseudo-dementia, agitated depressions, reactive depressions, neurotic depressions, masked depressions. This form of classification is based largely on a grouping

TABLE 3
SUMMARY OF CLINICAL MANIFESTATIONS OF DEPRESSION

1. Pervasive affect	Depressed, sad, crying spells; loss of interest and energy; exaggerated appearance of ageing
2. Physiological disturbances	Decreased and altered sleep patterns; decreased appetite and weight loss; constipation; tachycardia; pain – generalized or localized; gait abnormalities, tremors, rigidities
3. Psychological disturbances	Agitation, restlessness; retardation; confusion (difficulty in thinking, poor memory, unable to concentrate, temporary intellectual impairment); emptiness, hopelessness; dissatisfaction, personal devaluation; delusions; suicidal ruminations;

according to the dominant features of the depressive illness, and it has no special value in the overall management of the patient. It is perhaps more useful to distinguish between endogenous and reactive depression in older patients.

Endogenous and reactive depression
According to Post (1962) the majority of depressive illnesses in elderly people follow, within a few days, weeks or months, some outstanding occurrence in their lives. Thus two-thirds of his consecutively admitted depressives were 'reactive'. In 60% of the patients the precipitating events were: loss of health; loss of sources of affection (bereavement, serious illness of spouse, removal of children); loss of objects (retirement, moving from home, loss of property). The frequency of external events characterized by 'loss' increases with advancing age, and this may explain why the occurrence of the first onset of depression is often postponed to old age. Thus hereditary influences, although present, are less powerful in the depressions of later life. In Post's series 80% of the patients with the first attack of depression before the age of 50 had

TABLE 4
ENDOGENOUS AND REACTIVE DEPRESSION

	Endogenous	*Reactive*
Body build	Typically pyknic	Non-typical
Premorbid personality	Cyclothymic	Anxiety prone, hyper-sensitive
Precipitating factors	Proceeds independently of environmental stress	Environmental stress (a) situational; (b) physical illness
Depressive mood	Profound; unaffected by outside influences	Patchy; varies with out-side influences
Diurnal variation of mood	Worse in morning; im-proved by evening	Tired all day; often worse in evening
Sleep pattern	Early morning wakening	Difficulty in getting off to sleep
Blame	Tends to blame himself	Tends to blame others

a family history of depressive illness, compared with 44% in those patients with the first onset after the age of 65. Some of the points of distinction between endogenous and reactive depression are shown in Table 4.

Many of the features of the common type of reactive depression have been described by Wilson and Lawson (1962) under the heading 'situational depression'. They noted that among the admissions to a Geriatric Department there was a group of people who were miser-able, gloomy and taken up with themselves and their bodily com-plaints. There was no suicidal intent and they tend to blame their environmental and social situation for feelings that they would like to be dead. The patients generally had no feelings of guilt or self-reproach; they thought things had gone against them but they them-selves had done their best. The patients were nearly all widowed but living in comfortable circumstances, although they usually complained of great loneliness. There was often a feeling of hostility towards, and rejection by, the family. Three-quarters had life-long personality problems which however had not grossly affected their earlier lives. Many of the patients had marked physical disorders which rendered them bedridden. Depression responded rapidly after admission to hospital and long before the physical disorders were effectively treated. In fact, the relief of depression was due to the relief of physical symptoms in only one-third of cases, and it appears that non-specific aspects of geriatric care and the restoration of self-respect are the more imprortant therapeutic agents. These patients with situational depression, in contrast to those with endogenous or psychotic depression, are rarely seen by psychiatrists. Because the depression is associated with physical illness the condition is often first recognized by physicians in geriatric medicine.

Difficulties in recognition
In some elderly patients with depression, difficulties in diagnosis arise. Affective disorders are often unrecognized when mild, and there are no obvious changes in the appearance or behaviour of the patient. When patients present with an exacerbation of long-standing anxious, hypochondriacal or obsessional propensities they tend to be regarded as chronic neurotics who are becoming senile. At the other extreme severely disordered patients who are confused and inaccessible are often diagnosed as suffering from dementia. This is likely to be so when the patient becomes withdrawn, slowed up in actions and thought, tends to neglect himself or becomes very restless, with the result that a diagnosis is made of senile dementia and agitation. If marked persecutory symptoms are part of the clinical picture there may be a misdiagnosis of senile paraphenia or dementia with paranoid symptomatology.

Association with intellectual impairment
Many elderly patients appeared to be suffering from both depression and intellectual impairment, and there are several possible associations between the two:
   (1) Both depression and organic brain syndrome have a high incidence in old age and they can occur together by chance.

54

(2) Organic brain syndrome, especially multi-infarct dementia, like other physical illnesses may precipitate depression.

(3) Organic mental deterioration can lead to an inability to cope and to self-neglect in the home. The ensuing social isolation and adverse environmental situations are conductive to depression.

(4) Pseudo-dementia: this term describes the impairment of intellectual function resulting from depressive illness. Some of the ideational features of the depression are — difficulty in thinking, poor memory and inability to concentrate. Psychometric testing in these patients will show a temporary decline in cognitive function.

(5) Mental disorders are notable causes of malnutrition in old age, and in this respect depressive illness is more important than senile dementia (Exton-Smith, 1971). If there is a disinclination to obtain, prepare and even, in severe cases, to eat food, nutritional deficiencies may arise. Lack of thiamine, nicotinic acid and folic acid can cause acute or chronic confusional states.

A simple scoring system used for the assessment of mood, comparable to that used in the evaluation of intellectual function, would undoubtedly reveal many cases of depression in the elderly.

Treatment

In view of the association between depression and a variety of physical illnesses, the first essential for the proper management is a complete diagnosis. Underlying conditions should receive appropriate treatment, malnutrition should be corrected and severe constipation and faecal impaction should be relieved. Simple psychotherapy and the restoration of self-respect will often do much to help the patient with situational depression.

The tricyclic group of drugs is the most popular form of treatment for most cases of depression in the elderly. Imipramine can be given in an initial dose of 10 mg three times daily. Many patients will respond to this small dose but it can be increased to 25 mg three times a day after 2 weeks. Amitryptiline has a sedative effect and is indicated when depression is accompanied by anxiety, agitation and restlessness. The usual dose is 25 mg three times a day and this may conveniently be given as a single 75 mg dose at night. There is, however, a need to adjust the dose for each individual patient, since plasma levels may vary from 60μg/l to 600μg/l when amitryptiline is given in conventional therapeutic doses (Carr and Hobson, 1977); moreover failure of response to tricyclics occurs in cases with very low and very high plasma levels. Thus whenever the response is unsatisfactory it is advisable to measure the plasma levels as a guide to optimum dosage. Elderly patients treated with tricyclic antidepressants commonly develop adverse reactions, including blurring of vision, reduction of bowel motility with constipation and even adynamic ileus, retention of urine and postural hypotension. Some tricyclics induce serious cardiac arrhythmias which are believed to be due to an elevation of noradrenaline levels in heart tissue. There is some evidence that doxepin is less likely to be associated with arrhythmias and conduction defects, and the use of this drug is desirable in older patients with ECG abnormalities. L-tryptophan is sometimes a useful drug for treatment of depression in the elderly, particularly when associated with retardation. The use of monoamine-oxidase inhibitors (for example phenelzine) is rarely justified unless it is possible to supervise closely the drug and dietary regimens. The chief danger from their use is build-up of catecholamines causing hypertensive crises and intracranial haemorrhages when tyramine-rich foods (cheese, Marmite and broad beans) are eaten. Whenever there is a failure of response to adequate medication with antidepressant drugs the use of electro-convulsive therapy should be considered for all severly depressed elderly patients.

NEUROSIS

It has been estimated that approximately 12% of the elderly suffer from neurotic or personality disorders. Of these anxiety is the commonest.

Anxiety

Usually in the elderly there is a shift away from such symptoms of anxiety as sweating, tremor and palpitations to a more inward-looking, hypochondriacal concern that is often accompanied by depression (Post, 1962). Frequently this is triggered by a physical illness and leads to the patient expressing fear through numerous complaints.

There is often a background of an inadequate personality, poor relationships with the rest of the family and difficult social circumstances. Directing anxiety into fear of a specific situation or *phobia* may prevent the patient from travelling on the underground or being alone on a street, but is relatively uncommon in the elderly.

Hysteria

When used to mean an escape from anxiety through conversion into physical symptoms hysteria is rarely found in the elderly. If it does arise for the first time it should raise the possibility of an underlying depression.

Hypochondriasis

This is often a symptom of depression or anxiety, but sometimes represents a separate neurotic condition. Particularly in the elderly it may be an escape from personal failure.

Obsessional and compulsive behaviour

This rarely begins in old age but may persist from earlier life and worsen as the person becomes more inward-looking. Obsessional behaviour may be a feature of depression or dementia.

Management of the neuroses

The neurotic disorders do not respond readily to treatment. A patient,

57

understanding and supportive attitude is needed. The patient should be allowed to express his fears and concerns, if necessary over several interviews, and a detailed history should be taken of the social circumstances, family background and past history. Physical examination and reassurance are important but the patient cannot be fobbed off by telling him that there is nothing wrong. A minor tranquillizer may be prescribed and whenever possible the relatives should be seen, and an attempt made to relieve social stresses.

Hypochondriasis

The essential aim is to establish good rapport and so allow the patient to move from a recital of his physical complaints to an account of his social anxieties and stresses, with the hope that he may develop some insight (Busse and Pfeiffer, 1977). This takes patience and a good deal of time.

The physical complaints are a defence, and at no time must either the patient or his relatives feel that the doctor is dismissing them as 'emotional'. Prescriptions of a placebo, strictly timed interviews and a sympathetic hearing encourage the patient's trust.

PERSONALITY DISORDER

This is not a mental illness but means that the patient does not fit in harmoniously with the people around him and has probably been difficult and cantankerous all his life. He may prefer to go his own way, but problems arise when he can no longer maintain his independence and has to get on with others in hospital or a residential home. These unfortunate people tend to get hastily passed around between different institutions as everyone tries to unload the problem on to someone else.

It has to be recognized that there is little that can be done for such patients other than accept them as they are. This in itself may cause less acting up, and a tolerant attitude encourages the patient to settle down (Pitt, 1974). Moving the patient from one institution to another often aggravates antisocial behaviour and should be resisted.

Senile squalor syndrome

Occasionally an elderly person withdraws from society and becomes a recluse, hoarding all kinds of rubbish and living in filthy conditions. It is often difficult to get into their homes, not only because of the mountainous piles of belongings but because they resent interference.

This pattern has been described as the senile squalor syndrome (or Diogenes syndrome), and usually occurs in widows, living alone, whose personality is typically described as domineering, quarrelsome and independent (Macmillan and Shaw, 1966; Clark, Mannikar and Gray, 1975).

In most cases the patients are well known to social services but attempts to improve their condition are often rejected. Neighbours may demand that 'something must be done' because the situation offends their sense of what is right or because they are afraid of fire or vermin. Not uncommonly an acute illness leads to admission to hospital where the mortality, especially for women, is high.

Eccentricity and filthy habits alone are insufficient grounds for compulsory removal (under Section 47 of the National Assistance Act)* to a hospital or residential home. If a sane person has been offered help, refuses and subsequently dies of self-neglect, no legal blame attaches to anyone. However, one can try gentle persuasion and, particularly if an acte illness has meant hospital admission, recovery and the subsequent feeling of well-being and cleanliness may encourage the patient to accept a home help or day care. There is often a good response to day hospital support, though a great deal of tolerance by ambulance crew and nursing staff is needed initially.

ALCOHOLISM

The incidence in the UK among people over the age of 65 has been

---

* National Assistance Act of 1948 (Sec. 47) makes provision for compulsory admission of persons who: (a) are suffering from grave chronic disease, or, being aged, infirm or physically incapacitated, are living in insanitary conditions; and (b) are unable to devote to themselves, and are not receiving from other persons, proper care and attention.

estimated to be as high as 9%. Two-thirds of them are women. About half have been heavy drinkers all their lives with the rest starting to drink in old age as a symptom of reactive depression to stress or bereavement. Well-meaning relatives who are pleased to discover that their gift of a bottle of sherry or whisky is acceptable may, inadvertently, help a drinking habit to develop. Hospitalization is required so that accompanying physical disorders such as avitaminosis, skin sores, congestive cardiac failure and chronic bronchitis can be treated. The prospects for the patient remaning 'dry' depend very much on his willingness to admit that he has a problem, and the degree to which he will accept continuing support. Depression should be looked for and treated, and attempts made to find him some occupation such as in a sheltered workshop or day centre that he will find worthwhile.

PARANOIA

Paranoid reactions

These are commoner in old age than at other times of life, but are usually mild and transitory rather than disabling. Isolation and sensory deprivation increase with age so that hallucinations often fill in the emptiness and silence of the patient's life. Many such reactions are related to increasing deafness or failing vision.

Sometimes the patient blames others for his own failures and sees them as being hostile towards him. Usually it is a neighbour or relative who is accused of stealing, tampering with the walls or talking behind his back. These reactions are also seen in dementia, depression and occasionally as a side-effect of drugs such as steroids or L-dopa.

Paranoid psychoses (paraphrenia)

These are more serious, affect women much more than men and account for nearly 10% of elderly admissions to mental hospitals. The patients are approximately equally divided into those with a typical schizophrenic syndrome; those with paranoid delusions that are fairly understandable (such as being watched by a policeman); and those

60

TABLE 5
SIDE-EFFECTS OF PHENOTHIAZINES

1. Dizziness, drowsiness and postural hypotension
2. Disturbances of accommodation and bladder function
3. Extrapyramidal syndromes

3. Extrapyramidal syndromes
Parkinsonism ⎫
akathisia   ⎬ Early onset
dystonia   ⎭
tardive dyskinesia   Late onset

with auditory hallucinations alone (Post, 1966). They typically occur in women who live alone, are socially isolated and deaf. There is a significant association between paranoid psychoses and long-standing, severe, bilateral conductive deafness (Cooper and Curry, 1976).

TABLE 6
TARDIVE DYSKINESIA (Koch-Weser, 1977)

Features
Repetitive, involuntary movements of lips, tongue, head and limbs.
Occur with increasing frequency with age.
Associated with prolonged use and high doses of antipsychotic drugs.
May appear at any time during treatment but especially after antipsychotic treatment stopped.
Due to denervation hypersensitivity caused by chronic dopamine receptor blockade.

Prevention
Avoid long-term, high-dose antipsychotic drugs if possible.
'Drug holidays' to unmask dyskinesia.
Stop antipsychotic drugs at first sign of dyskinesia.

Treatment
Unsatisfactory. Aim to reduce brain dopamine or block dopamine receptors.
Try tetrabenazine (initially 25 twice daily) or pimozide (initially 2 mg three times daily).

Management

The patient is helped by a calm, sympathetic approach. If the psychosis is severe she should be admitted to hospital. A phenothiazine such as thioridazine (25 mg three times daily and 50 mg nocte, although much higher doses may be needed) is effective and has a minimum of extrapyramidal side-effects (see Table 5). A monthly intramuscular injection of fluphenazine decanoate (25–50 mg after a small, initial test dose) is useful when the patient cannot be relied upon to take her drugs. If tremor, muscle stiffness and excessive salivation are troublesome then benzhexol (2–6 mg daily in divided doses) may be added. However the routine prescribing of an anticholinergic drug with a phenothiazine should be avoided since anticholinergics may worsen or even induce tardive dyskinesias (see Table 6). Spectacles and a hearing aid may be needed.

REFERENCES

Botez, M. I., Ethier, R., Léveillé, J. and Botez-Marquard, T. (1977). A syndrome of early recognition of occult hydrocephalus and cerebral atrophy. *Q. J. Med.*, NS, **46,** 365

Bowen, D. M. and Davison, A. N. (1978). Biochemical changes in the normal ageing brain and in dementia. In B. Isaacs (ed.). *Recent Advances in Geriatric Medicine* (Edinburgh: Churchill Livingstone)

Busse, E. W. and Pfeiffer, E. (1977). Functional psychiatric disorders in old age. In *Behaviour and Adaptation in Late Life*. 2nd. ed. (Boston: Little, Brown and Co.)

Carr, A. C. and Hobson, R. P. (1977). High serum concentrations of antidepressants in the elderly patients. *Br. Med. J.*, **2,** 1151

Clark, A. N. G., Mannikar, G. D. and Gray, I. (1975). Diogenes syndrome: a clinical study of gross neglect in old age. *Lancet*, **i,** 366

Cooper, A. F. and Curry, A. R. (1976). The pathology of deafness in the paranoid and affective psychoses of later life. *J. Psychosom. Res.*, **20,** 97

Dalziel, J. A. and Griffiths, R. A. (1977). Progressive supranuclear palsy. *Age and Ageing*, **6,** 185

Davis, K. L., Mohs, R. C., Tinklenberg, J. R. Pfefferbaum, A., Hollister, L. E. and Kopell, B. S. (1978). Physostigmine: improvement of long term memory processes in normal humans. *Science*, **201**, 272

Drachman, D. A and Leavitt, J. (1974). Human memory and the cholinergic system: a relationship to ageing? *Arch. Neurol.*, **30**, 113

Dronefield, M. W., Mead, G. M. and Langman, M. J. S. (1977). Survival and death from subdural haematoma on medical wards. *Postgrad. Med. J.*, **53**, 57

Exton-Smith, A. N. (1971). Nutrition of the elderly, *Br. J. Hosp. Med.*, **5**, 639

Hachinski, V. C. Lassen, N. A. and Marshall, J. (1974). Multi-infarct dementia. A cause of mental deterioration in the elderly. *Lancet*, **ii**, 207

Hachinski, V. C., Iliff, L. D., Zilkha, E., Du Boulay, G. H., Mcallister, V. L., Marshall, J., Ross Russell, R. W. and Symon, L. (1975). Cerebral blood flow in dementia. *Arch. Neurol*, **32**, 632

Holden, U. P. and Sinebruchow, A. (1978). Reality orientation therapy: a study investigating the value of this therapy in the rehabilitation of elderly people. *Age and Ageing*, **7**, 83

Hyams, D. E. (1978). Cerebral function and drug therapy. In J. C. Brocklehurst (ed.). *Textbook of Geriatric Medicine and Gerontology*. 2nd edn. (Edinburgh: Churchill Livingstone)

Kay, D. W. K., Beamish, P. and Roth, M. (1964). Old age mental disorders in Newcastle upon Tyne. *Br. J. Psych.*, **110**, 146

Koch-Weser, J. (1977). Drug therapy of tardive dyskinesia. *N. Engl. J. Med.*, **296**, 257

Macmillan, D. and Shaw, P. (1966). Senile breakdown in standards of personal and environmental cleanliness. *Br. Med. J.*, **2**, 1032

Marsden, C. D. and Harrison, M. J. G. (1972). Outcome of investigation of patients with presenile dementia. *Br. Med. J.*, **2**, 249

Pitt, B. (1974). *Psychogeriatrics: an Introduction to the Psychiatry of Old Age*. (Edinburgh: Churchill Livingstone)

Post, F. (1962) *The Significance of Affective Symptoms in Old Age*. (London: Oxford University Press)

Post, F. (1965). *The Clinical Psychiatry of Later Life*. (Oxford: Pergamon Press)

Post, F. (1966). *Persistent Persecutory States of the Elderly*. (Oxford: Pergamon Press)

Roth, M. and Myers, D. H. (1969). The diagnosis of dementia. *Br. J. Hosp. Med.*, **2**, 705

Signoret, J. L. Whiteley, A. and Lhermitte, F. (1978). Influence of choline on amnesia in early Alzheimer's disease. *Lancet*, **ii**, 837

Sitaram, N., Weingarten, H. and Gillin, J. C. (1978). Human serial learning: enhancement with arecoline and choline and impairment with scopolamine. *Science,* **201,** 274

Spillane, J. A., White, P., Goodhardt, M. J., Flack, R. H. A., Bowen, D. M. and Davison, A. N. (1977). Selective vulnerability of neurones in organic dementia. *Nature,* **226,** 558

Strub, R. L. and Black, F. W. (1977); *The Mental Status Examination in Neurology.* (Philadelphia: F. A. Davis Co.)

White, P., Hiley, C. R., Goodhardt, M. J., Carrasco, L. H., Keet, J. P., Williams, I. E. I. and Bowen, D. M. (1977). Neocortical cholinergic neurones in elderly people. *Lancet,* **i,** 668

Wilson, L. A. and Lawson, I. R. (1962). Situational depression in the elderly. *Gerontol. Clin. Addit. Ad.,* **4,** 59

4
Central nervous system and special senses

The clinical presentation of neurological disorders in old age is frequently influenced by age-related changes in the central nervous system. These changes may be intrinsic and part of the process of ageing (see Chapter 3) or they may be the result of pathological conditions in other organs and tissues, especially in the cardiovascular system. Critchley (1931) has drawn attention to the effects of ageing on neurological signs. Many physical signs indicative of disease in the young may not be of significance in the diagnosis of clinical neurological disorders in old age. Thus loss of vibration sense and tendon jerks in the lower limbs do not necessarily mean peripheral neuropathy; irregular sluggish pupils are not pathognomonic of neurosyphilis and the frequent occurrence of a bodily attitude of flexion, disorders of gait, tremors and a positive glabellar tap sign leads to difficulties in establishing the diagnosis of Parkinsonism.

A large number of neurological disorders which are encountered in old age can be attributed directly to changes in the arterial blood supply to the brain. In addition to being one of the commonest causes

65

of morbidity and mortality in old age, cerebrovascular disease is the biggest single physical cause of hospital-bed occupancy by the elderly in the United Kingdom (Hunt, 1973). Stroke illness accounts for 20% of the bed occupancy; heart and blood vessel diseases (excluding strokes) 16%, and malignant disease 8%. A stroke is only one of several presentations of cerebral vascular disease, but the rehabilitation of the patient with a completed stroke forms one of the commonest clinical problems in geriatric practice.

STROKE

A stroke is defined as an acute disturbance of cerebral function of presumed vascular origin with disability lasting more than 24 hours. This definition excludes temporary disturbances of function (transient ischaemic attacks), multi-infarct dementia, and manifestations simulating those of a stroke due to cerebral tumour. The incidence of stroke rises steeply with age, from approximately 3 per 1000 in those aged 55–64 to 8 per 1000 aged 65–74 and to 25 per 1000 in people aged 75 and over. The sexes are about equally affected and about 130 000 people in the United Kingdom at any one time suffer appreciable ill health because they have had one or more strokes (Harris, Cox and Smith, 1971).

Causes

The two most important vascular causes of stroke are cerebral infarction and cerebral haemorrhage. The former is responsible for nearly three-quarters and the latter nearly one-quarter of the cases. It is appropriate to use the term 'cerebral infarction' to include cerebral thrombosis and cerebral embolism. In the past the importance of cerebral embolism has been underestimated and it is now believed to be responsible for 45% of cases of cerebral infarction (Blackwood *et al.*, 1969).

Cerebral infarction
This is commonly due to arterial occlusion by atheroma, thrombosis

and embolism. The distribution of atheroma is often patchy and tends to affect particular arteries at certain sites. Hypertension is an important predisposing cause contributing to the severity of atherosclerosis. In some cases cerebral infarction occurs in the absence of occlusion of the main vessels, for example, when there is systemic hypotension due to cardiac infarction or gastrointestinal haemorrhage. Even more important it has been known for many years that the cerebral artery supplying the infarcted area is often still patent; in these cases the occlusion is to be found in the proximal parts of the carotid or vertebral arteries in the neck (Fisher, 1954; Hutchinson and Yates, 1957). Lesions in these arteries can be a source of emboli which occlude the cerebral vessels to cause infarction, and they consist of friable mixtures of platelets and debris from atheromatous lesions; these may break up too soon to be detected by arteriography or at post-mortem examination. Embolism may occur from a fibrillating left atrium especially in mitral stenosis.

Cerebral haemorrhage
This is usually the result of rupture of perforating arteries in hypertensive patients, and occurs mainly in the basal ganglia and less comonly in the mid-brain, brain stem and cerebellum. Other causes of haemorrhage are rupture of microaneurysms (Charcot–Bouchard type) and of berry aneurysms. The collection of blood may be localized in the brain to form a haematoma, but in 80% of cases blood is present in the cerebrospinal fluid.

Clinical features

The neurological manifestations of cerebrovascular accident are many and diverse, according to the site, type and extent of spread, and speed of development of the vascular lesion. Thus the presentation may range from an abrupt onset and rapid evolution of hemiplegia with loss of consciousness to a gradual cumulative change in the neurological picture over many months. The territory supplied by the middle cerebral artery is most often involved.

Disorder of motor function

Initially there may be flaccid paralysis with loss of reflexes on the hemiplegic side. With the development of hypertonicity on the affected side the arm is internally rotated and adducted at the shoulder and the wrist and fingers are flexed. The leg is usually in extension with marked loss of power of dorsiflexion at the ankle joint. This is the usual picture of middle cerebral artery or carotid artery occlusion and the loss of power is greater in the arm than in the leg. If the anterior cerebral artery is involved the loss of power in the upper limb is minimal, affecting shoulder joint movements, and in the leg the loss of power is most marked distally, and involves mainly movements of the foot.

Disturbances of sensation

Cortical and subcortical lesions in the parietal lobe lead to hemianaesthesia and to sensory neglect on the affected side. Sensory impairment is more marked distally and affects particularly the spatial and discriminative aspects of sensation. Thus there may be astereognosis and impaired two-point discrimination as well as sensory ataxia due to impaired position sense in the affected limbs. If the proximal parts of the limbs and trunk are involved the anaesthesia does not extend quite to the midline. Parietal lobe manifestations are most often found in non-dominant hemisphere lesions; they should always be sought initially by simultaneous bilateral stimulation of the limbs and later confirmed by more sophisticated tests of sensory function. They always present a serious handicap to recovery, especially when there is a disturbance of the body image, lack of awareness of the affected limbs or denial of disability (anosognosia). The parietal lobe lesion in the dominant hemisphere may give rise to Gerstmann's syndrome characterized by left–right disorientation, finger agnosia, agraphia, acalculia and constructional apraxia.

Visual disturbances

Involvement of the optic radiation gives rise to homonymous hemianopia affecting the field of vision on the side of the paralysed limbs.

This too leads to difficulty in rehabilitation, especially when a parietal lobe lesion leads to neglect of the left half of the external space (unilateral visual agnosia). This can be demonstrated by the simultaneous bilateral presentation of visual stimuli and by asking the patient to insert the figures in a circle to represent a clock face.

Aphasia

Disturbances of language and communication due to aphasia (dysphasia) occur in about two-thirds of cases of right hemiplegia in the series reported by Marquardsen (1969). This author also showed that aphasic patients have a higher mortality and poorer prognosis with regard to functional recovery than patients with comparable physical disability but with no language disturbance. There have been many attempts to classify aphasia but here it will serve to mention the simplest classification.

Mainly expressive aphasia   This consists of an inability to express ideas through written and spoken speech. Comprehension is often good. In its less severe form the dysphasia is nominal and the patient has difficulty in selecting the correct word.

Mainly receptive aphasia   In this condition there is impairment of understanding or oral and graphic symbols. Some of these patients have jargon aphasia.

Total aphasia   Total aphasia leads to absence of communication by speaking, writing and reading. In rare cases the patient has a single or recurring utterance.

Apraxia

This condition results from a disorder of integrative action within the nervous system, and consists of an inability to carry out purposive movements in the absence of severe paralysis, ataxia or sensory loss. It is usually most obvious in the upper limb with difficulty in carrying out skilled actions with the hand.

69

Mental symptoms and disturbed behaviour

Cerebral damage which is responsible for hemiplegia often leads to reduction in intellectual capacity and impairment of memory. With extensive brain damage especially when there are vascular lesions elsewhere in the brain the mental deterioration amounts to dementia. Some patients show a catastrophic reaction in which there is a sudden change from amiable cooperation to outbursts of aggression and anti-social behaviour. Emotional instability with a tendency to laughter and tears without apparent cause is also common. Loss of physical capacity due to hemiplegia is an important cause of situational depression (see Chapter 3).

Incontinence

Incontinence of urine commonly results from loss of cortical inhibition of spontaneous bladder contractions. In the uninhibited neurogenic bladder the musculature is hypertonic and hyperexcitable. Cystometrographic studies in hemiplegic patients show detrusor instability, but the characteristics are similar to those found in many other incontinent patients without hemiplegia.

Epilepsy

Convulsions appearing for the first time in old age are very likely to be due to cerebrovascular disease. They may be either focal or generalized. Marquardsen (1969) found that about 5% of patients who had recovered from a stroke later developed epilepsy, and in two-thirds of these the onset was within 2 years of the cerebral catastrophe. Paroxysmal pain in the hemiplegic limbs is sometimes an epileptic phenomenon and this may respond to anticonvulsant therapy.

Pseudobulbar palsy

The corticospinal tracts are damaged on both sides by bilateral lesions involving the basal ganglia, the thalamus and the internal capsules. The onset may appear to be sudden but there have usually been some premonitory signs. The main features consist of paresis of the face, the palate and the pharynx with difficulties in mastication and

70

deglutition. The dysarthria gives rise to a nasal type of speech. On account of pharyngeal weakness there is difficulty in swallowing liquids which may be regurgitated through the nose. Attacks of uncontrollable crying or laughing without adequate provocation are characteristic. Impairment of intellectual faculties is common. There is evidence of bilateral pyramidal tract damage, but the signs vary. Some patients show hemiplegia with pseudobulbar symptoms, some show paraplegia, whilst others have severe bulbar symptoms without evidence of weakness of the limbs.

Diagnosis

The probable anatomical location of the stroke lesion can usually be determined on clinical grounds, but the pathological differentiation of infarction from haemorrhage is often inaccurate without fuller investigation. Clinical features favouring the diagnosis of haemorrhage are: an onset with severe headache, vomiting, or immediate loss of consciousness, signs of rapid progression of the lesion, stiffness of the neck, conjugate deviation of the eyes and abnormalities in the depth, rate and rhythm of respiration. The diagnostic procedures used in the investigation of strokes are shown in Table 1. Some of these procedures are of limited value, but in general the more investigations carried out, particularly if a CAT scan is included, the more accurate the diagnosis will be.

Besides the differentiation of infarction and haemorrhage it is also necessary to exclude a number of less common causes of stroke.

Cerebral tumour
Post-mortem examination and more recently CAT show that cerebral tumour is present in about 10% of cases diagnosed as suffering from cerebrovascular strokes.

Myocardial infarction
In about 2% of patients with acute myocardial infarction the presenting feature is a stroke. Thompson and Robinson (1978) have shown that the likelihood of a stroke is related to the infarct size. When the

71

TABLE 1
INVESTIGATIONS IN STROKE

Procedure	Value – limitations
Echo-encephalography	will reveal midline shift but this will occur in both cerebral infarction and haemorrhage
Electroencephalography	reflects the size and location of the lesion rather than its pathological cause
Brain scan	isotope uptake excessive in haemorrhage and infarcts; returns to normal within a few weeks, but not in tumours
Lumbar puncture	presence of blood in CSF indicates haemorrhage, but absent in 20% cases of cerebral haemorrhage
Cerebral angiography	will reveal stenosis, occlusion of vessels, aneurysms and tumour; limited use in patients over 70
Computerized axial tomography (CAT)	most accurate method of demonstrating intra-cerebral haemorrhage and its differentiation from infarction or tumour (in some cases difficult to distinguish infarct from tumour)

peak level of creatine kinase (CK) was in the upper third of the range of values (above 1160 iu/l) the incidence of stroke was 24 times the incidence when the peak CK was below this level. Electro-cardiography is an essential investigation in all patients with strokes, not only to detect a possible underlying cause of stroke but also be-cause coexistent myocardial ischaemia may be a limiting factor in rehabilitation.

Subdural haematoma
This condition should be suspected when the degree of hemiparesis is mild in relation to the level of consciousness, especially when this level shows fluctuations.

Giant cell arteritis
Involvement of intracerebral vessels should be suspected in the eld-erly patient with stroke who has progressive cerebral ischaemia, a

high ESR and complains of headache, even in the absence of inflamed temporal arteries.

Drug-induced hypoglycaemia

Persistent hypoglycaemia resulting from the use of long-acting anti-diabetic agents such as chlorpropamide may produce a clinical condition simulating stroke in the elderly (Schen and Benaroya, 1976).

Prognosis

The immediate prognosis depends on the nature and extent of the underlying lesion. It is worse in cerebral haemorrhage than in infarction; nearly three-quarters of patients with cerebral haemorrhage are dead within 6 months compared with less than half of those with cerebral infarction. The prognosis is also worse when embolism is the basis of infarction, but precise evaluation is difficult owing to the problems of the accurate differentiation of embolic and thrombotic occlusion. Oxbury and his colleagues (1975) have shown a relationship between level of consciousness on admission and outcome in cerebral infarction; in the first 3 weeks there was no mortality in those who were fully conscious, but one-third of those who were drowsy or confused, and one-half of those who were unresponsive or unconscious, had died within the same period. In patients who had complete paralysis of the upper and lower limb the mortality was three times as great as those who had some movement in the limbs.

The long-term prognosis as regards functional recovery depends not only on the degree of motor paralysis but also on other effects of cerebral damage which form part of the stroke syndrome, such as impaired control of movement, disorders of vision and perception especially in parietal lobe involvement, disturbances of cognition and the presence of aphasia (see page 69). Elderly patients with stroke have a high incidence of coexisting coronary and hypertensive heart disease and of peripheral vascular disease, and Marquardsen (1969) has shown that the ultimate prognosis in stroke is determined by that of the accompanying disease. Common causes of death due to these generalized vascular changes are cardiac failure, pulmonary embolism, recurrence of stroke and myocardial infarction.

Treatment

There are usually two phases in the management of the patient who has suffered a stroke. In the first phase, immediately after the onset good nursing and expert medical care are essential. Later treatment depends on specific measures to improve function; these aspects of rehabilitation are discussed in Chapter 15.

At present the emergency treatment of stroke has little to offer. Patients with intracerebral haemorrhage, confirmed on CAT scanning, can sometimes be treated by surgical evacuation of the haematoma. The value of treatment purported to reduce oedema in cerebral infarction is now in doubt. Mulley, Wilcox and Mitchell (1978) showed no difference in the number of survivors and in the quality of life at 1 year in a controlled trial of immediate treatment with dexamethasone in patients with acute stroke. Llarsson, Marinovich and Barber (1976) were unable to uphold the claim of dramatic improvement in stroke patients treated with an intravenous infusion of glycerol. In view of the lack of specific treatment the need for admission of the stroke patient to hospital has been questioned. There are, however, advantages in hospital admission as Mulley and Arie (1978) have pointed out; important amongst these are the need to make an accurate diagnosis to exclude the rarer and sometimes treatable causes, and to make a precise assessment of all the disabilities. Although treatment of patients in an acute stroke unit may not reduce overall mortality, skilled treatment in the early stages can reduce the incidence of complications.

TRANSIENT ISCHAEMIC ATTACKS

Transient cerebral ischaemic attacks (TIAs) are defined as the sudden occurrence of usually repeated episodes of sensory or motor impairment caused by temporary inadequacy of blood flow to a localized area of the brain and disappearing completely within 24 hours. It is the manifestations which should be regarded as transient, since the underlying pathological process is usually a progressive disease, atheroma, affecting the large and medium-sized arteries.

Aetiology

There are several precipitating causes of TIAs. The most important is the production of microemboli from platelet aggregates in atheromatous ulcers. On account of laminar flow in the cerebral vessels these multiple emboli tend to produce a series of TIAs which have a stereotyped pattern. The second important cause is a transient cardiac dysrhythmia, often a short burst of tachycardia, which is usually only recognized by 24-hour electrocardiographic monitoring (prolonged tape-recorded ECG shows transient dysrhythmia in 20% of patients suffering from TIAs). Fall in cerebral blood flow occurs in postural hypotension (see Chapter 5) and in myocardial infarction, especially in elderly subjects whose control of cerebral autoregulation is impaired. Cervical spondylosis, which interferes with flow in the vertebral arteries, is an important factor causing vertebrobasilar TIAs. Additional predisposing causes are anaemia, which reduces the oxygen-carrying capacity of the blood, and polycythaemia, which reduces cerebral blood flow by increasing the viscosity of the blood.

Clinical features

The onset of a TIA is usually sudden, the attack lasts a few minutes and the symptoms then gradually subside. When the carotid territory is involved the manifestation is usually a transient hemiparesis; there may in addition be hemianopia, numbness in the affected limbs and dysphasia in a dominant hemisphere lesion. In vertebrobasilar TIAs the features include transient vertigo and ataxia, dysarthria, dysphagia, parasthesiae over the face and hemiplegia. Drop attacks (see page 87) may also be a manifestation of vertebrobasilar insufficiency.

TIAs carry a greatly increased risk of subsequent stroke; one-third to one-half of the patients develop a stroke within 5 years of the initial attack.

Treatment

Although the use of anticoagulants will reduce the likelihood of subsequent TIAs and a subsequent stroke in the elderly, control is difficult and their use tends to be restricted to patients who can be very closely supervised; even then there is a higher risk of complications. Another approach has been the use of drugs which inhibit platelet aggregation. A cooperative trial in Canada (1978) has shown in 585 patients with TIAs who were followed for 26 months that aspirin (600 mg daily) reduced the risk of stroke or death by 48% in the men; there was no benefit for the women. Sulphinpyrazone produced a small reduction in stroke and death, but this was not statistically significant. Thus in men when it can be ascertained that the source of microemboli is an atheromatous plaque which cannot be treated surgically by endarterectomy the use of aspirin prophylactically offers the best prospects. When prolonged electrocardiographic monitoring shows cardiac dysrhythmias these should be treated by the appropriate drugs or by the insertion of a pacemaker.

PARKINSONISM

Paralysis agitans, or the 'shaking palsy', was first described by James Parkinson in 1817. It is a disorder characterized by tremor, muscular rigidity and slowness, weakness and poverty of movement. The incidence rises steeply after the age of 50 and in the United Kingdom it occurs in about 1.5% of the population over the age of 60.

Aetiology

The main forms of Parkinsonism are:

Idiopathic
Paralysis agitans or Parkinson's disease in which the main disorder

76

of function is in the extrapyramidal system, although autonomic disturbances occur in many cases.

Post-encephalitic

Parkinsonism is seen in the survivors of the pandemic of encephalitis lethargica which occurred after World War I. Clinical manifestations of damage in other parts of the nervous system may be present.

Cerebrovascular

Multi-infarct disease leads to Parkinsonian features with bradykinesia and rigidity more conspicuous than tremor. There are usually associated features of focal pyramidal tract damage, pseudobulbar palsy or dementia.

Drug-induced

Drugs may produce Parkinsonism by preventing the action of dopamine on the brain. Phenothiazines and butyrophenones (e.g. haloperidol) block the post-synaptic dopamine receptors, and reserpine and tetrabenazine prevent dopamine release from the presynaptic neurones.

Other cerebral disorders which may give rise to Parkinson's syndrome include progressive supranuclear palsy, the Shy–Drager syndrome, olivo-pontocerebellar degeneration and Jakob–Creutzfeld disease (see Chapters 3 and 5). In Alzheimer's disease (presenile and senile dementia) mild features of Parkinsonism occur in association with widespread brain atrophy.

Pathogenesis

The most constant pathological finding is the loss of pigmented neurones in the substantia nigra; less often there is a reduction of small nerve cells in the globus pallidus. Recently it has been shown (Hakim and Mathieson, 1978) that generalized cerebral atrophy occurs to a greater extent than would be expected for the patient's age, and there is an increase in the numbers of neurofibrillary tangles and senile plaques. There is thus an overlap between Parkinsonism and Alzheimer's disease.

Neurochemical investigations of the brains of Parkinsonian patients show a deficiency of dopamine in the nigrostriatal pathway. The severity of akinesia is correlated significantly with the degree of dopamine deficiency found in the caudate nucleus. This, however, is not the sole explanation of the clinical features since concurrently there is a relative excess of cholinergic neurotransmission and brain biochemical studies show an increase in the ratio of acetylcholinesterase to dopamine. Clinically, anticholinergic agents produce worthwhile improvement in some patients.

The disease process itself is unaltered by dopamine replacement in spite of a good early therapeutic response. This has been attributed to the progressive loss of dopamine receptors in the caudate nucleus; indeed the changes of chronic denervation may lead to hypersensitivity at the receptor sites with the occurrence of dyskinetic syndromes in patients treated for long periods with levodopa. These syndromes are especially common in elderly Parkinsonian patients whose brains have undergone diffuse atrophy. Thus imbalance between cholinergic and dopaminergic activities is only one of the disturbed mechanisms in Parkinsonism, and it is likely that other neurotransmitters are involved such as gamma-aminobutyric acid (GABA), noradrenaline and serotonin.

Clinical picture

The general features of Parkinsonism present a distinctive picture. The symptoms and signs can be grouped as follows:

Appearance
Immobility of facial muscles leads to an impassive facial expression. There is diminished blinking and eye movements with widening of the palpebral fissures. The general body posture is one of slight to moderate flexion and the limbs are flexed and adducted at proximal joints.

78

The fingers are flexed at the metacarpophalangeal joints and extended distally with the thumb adducted and extended.

Voluntary movement

Weakness affects particularly the small muscles: articulatory muscles – speech slow, slurred and monotonous; oculomotor muscles – weak convergence; jaw and pharyngeal muscles – slow mastication and difficulty in swallowing; fine finger movements – difficulty in writing, sewing, etc. Slowness of movement is often a more marked feature than weakness. An early sign results from impairment of associated synergic movements with absence of swinging the arms on walking, and gestures accompanying speech. Inability to initiate movement (akinesia) leads to difficulty in turning in bed, getting up from a chair and in commencing to walk.

Involuntary movement

The tremor, consisting of rhythmical movements at the rate of four to six per second, is most conspicuous at rest and is diminished on voluntary movement and during sleep. It usually begins unilaterally in an arm and extends to the lower limb on the same side before involving the opposite arm. The rhythmic flexion and extension of the metacarpophalangeal joints with adduction of the thumb, is responsible for the classical pill-rolling movements.

Muscular rigidity

The agonists and antagonists are uniformly affected with the characteristic 'lead-pipe' rigidity. In the presence of tremor the rigidity is of the 'cog-wheel' type. When rigidity is severe contractures develop and these further restrict movement.

Gait

Bradykinesia leads to a shuffling gait with short steps. With increasing flexion and diminished control of equilibrium the patient develops a 'festinant' gait as if trying to catch up with his centre of gravity. There may be difficulty in initiating walking and in changing direction.

Falls
The patient with Parkinsonism has a marked tendency to fall, due to several causes, including tripping associated with the shuffling gait, difficulty in restoring equilibrium once it has been disturbed, and when postural hypotension is present to impairment of cerebral blood flow.

Autonomic disturbances
The commonest autonomic disturbance is excessive salivation; other manifestations are cutaneous vasodilatation with undue feeling of warmth, impaired temperature regulation and the hazards of hypothermia and postural hypotension (see Chapter 5).

Mental changes
Some elderly patients with Parkinsonism show early features of typical Alzheimer-type dementia (Hakim and Mathieson, 1978). Confusional states are liable to develop in response to infection such as bronchopneumonia (Hodkinson, 1973) or to drugs used in treatment. Depression is also a common psychiatric disorder.

Diagnosis

It is sometimes difficult to differentiate the early stages of Parkinsonism from the physiological changes in posture and movement which accompany normal ageing (see Chapter 2). It is also necessary to distinguish Parkinsonism from:

(1) *Senile tremor* which affects the head more than the limbs; it is faster than Parkinsonian tremor and is induced by movement; there is no associated bradykinesia, muscle weakness or rigidity.
(2) *Conditions associated with rigidity*, such as progressive supranuclear palsy, Shy–Drager syndrome and pseudobulbar palsy.

(3) *Alzheimer-type dementia* in which features of mild Parkinsonism are present. Examination should include the elicitation of primitive (snout and palmo-mental) reflexes.

Prognosis

Although the main identifiable biochemical abnormality, dopamine deficiency, is now amenable to treatment, the prime cause remains unknown. There is no evidence that the progressive course of the disease can be influenced by therapy. Nevertheless, treatment with levodopa and related drugs usually improves the symptoms and prolongs the period in which the patient can remain physically independent. Thus the dangers of the bedridden state (contractures, bedsores, pneumonia and thromboembolism) are often delayed or averted. With effective drug therapy more deaths are due to trauma, accidental falls, fractures (especially the femoral neck) and unrelated conditions.

Treatment

The basis of treatment is to correct the imbalance between the dopaminergic and cholinergic systems. Whatever form of therapy is used side-effects are common and these can sometimes be reduced by a combination of drugs. It is also important in the elderly to start with small doses, to increase the doses by small increments and at long intervals with careful titration to the individual needs of the patient.

Dopaminergic agents
Dopamine itself will not cross the blood–brain barrier, but its precursor, levodopa, does so readily.

Levodopa This should be started in a dose of 250 mg once or twice daily after meals and gradually increased by 125 mg twice weekly to a final level of about 2 g daily within a period of 6–8 weeks. Improvement in akinesia, bradykinesia and tremor can be expected in about 70% of patients.

Carbidopa combined with levodopa (Sinemet) Can be used to reduce the dosage of levodopa. Carbidopa is an inhibitor which does not pass the blood–brain barrier; it reduces the decarboxylation of levodopa in the peripheral tissues and enables more levodopa to reach the striatum. It is available as 25 mg carbidopa combined with 250 mg levodopa or as 10 mg carbidopa with 100 mg levodopa. The smaller dosage is usually more appropriate for elderly patients.

Bromocriptine Bromocriptine is a dopamine agonist. When given alone it has no advantages over levodopa, and it is best used in patients where initial response to levodopa is good but who later develop the on–off phenomenon. The combination of bromocriptine (20–40 mg daily) and levodopa allows the dosage of levodopa to be reduced and often confers benefit by producing a smoother action.

The side-effects of levodopa and other dopaminergic drugs include:

- (i) Nausea and vomiting which can sometimes be controlled with metoclopramide 10–30 mg daily (phenothiazine anti-emetics must not be used).
- (ii) Orthostatic hypotension – treatment must usually be stopped or dosage reduced.
- (iii) Cardiac arrhythmias can often be controlled with propranolol.
- (iv) Dyskinetic syndromes occur especially in the elderly.
- (v) 'On–off' phenomenon consisting of day-to-day fluctuations in the response which swings from activity to immobility.
- (vi) Mental disturbances – hallucinations, paranoid delusions and depression.

Anticholinergic agents
Many patients still derive benefit from these drugs either alone or in combination with levodopa. Those most often used are benzhexol, benztropine mesylate, benapyrazine, procyclidine and orphenadrine. They produce slight improvement in tremor, moderate reduction in

rigidity and often useful control of excessive salivation. Elderly patients are especially at risk of developing side-effects including mental confusion, hallucinations, blurred vision and urinary retention.

Other drugs

Amantadine is believed to act by release of dopamine from intact dopaminergic terminals. When given in doses of 100 mg two or three times a day it enables the dosage of levodopa given concurrently to be reduced. L-deprenyl is a selective inhibitor of monoamine oxidase type B, and may increase the available dopamine at receptor sites by inhibiting its breakdown (Lees *et al.*, 1977). It may be useful in decreasing the 'on–off' phenomenon.

General management

Advantage must be taken of the good response to drug therapy by means of a systematic programme of rehabilitation. Physiotherapy and occupational therapy will be required regularly both for inpatients and outpatients. The procedures involved are practice in turning in bed, getting in and out of a chair, dressing and bathing, walking exercises and the correction of abnormal postures by postural and balance exercises before a mirror. Gratifying improvement can often be achieved even with advanced disability, but the main limiting factors in improvement are the side-reactions to drug therapy and the mental deterioration due to Alzheimer-like changes associated with cerebral atrophy.

CERVICAL SPONDYLOSIS

On the basis of X-ray changes, cervical spondylosis is almost universal by the age of 70 but the relation between symptoms and X-ray changes is poor. Brain (1963) reported on 100 patients with cervical spondylosis and found that the commonest presenting symptoms were brachial radiculitis (32%), headache (28%), giddiness (17%), vertebrobasilar insufficiency (5%), attacks of unconsciousness (4%)

and drop attacks (3%).

Cervical spondylosis frequently coexists with atheroma involving the vertebral and basilar arteries, and in such cases it may reduce still further the already poor vertebrobasilar circulation and produce giddiness, diplopia, facial sensory disturbance, dysarthria etc. In addition to causing brain-stem signs through compression of the vertebral artery, cervical spondylosis may also produce a myelopathy and spastic weakness of the legs which will contribute to the patient's unsteadiness.

However, the association between cervical spondylosis and postural imbalance is a complex one, and it is only fairly recently that the importance of cervical articular mechanoreceptor function has been recognized (Wyke, 1979). There are, in the layers of the fibrous capsule of each cervical joint, two types of receptors: type I which are excited by the stresses inherent in sitting or standing still, and type II which are stimulated only by movements of the neck. The tonic afferent discharges from these receptors produce a complex series of reflex changes in the muscles of the neck, suboccipital region, jaw, eye and all four limbs. These are powerful reflexes, as can be shown in decerebrate cats by the coordinated movements of all four limbs produced by passive rotation of the head on the neck: a phenomenon which can be utilized in helping hemiplegic patients to walk. Significantly, the function of these cervical mechanoreceptors declines with age and the decline is accelerated by inflammatory or degenerative cervical joint disease. Thus it is probable that poor mechanoreceptor function is responsible for an appreciable amount of postural imbalance in the elderly. Furthermore experimental impairment of cervical mechanoreceptor function will produce vertigo, nystagmus and arm apraxia – symptoms which are very similar to those produced by vertebrobasilar insufficiency. Presumably some patients are misdiagnosed as having poor vertebrobasilar blood flow when in fact the disorder lies in their cervical joints.

Treatment

Patients who have brachial radiculitis or vertebrobasilar insufficiency proven on angiography, and which is aggravated by cervical spondy-losis, may have a trial in a cervical collar. This must fit well, hold the spine in slight flexion and be worn night and day, but for no longer than 3 months (Storey, 1971). However, there is no evidence that the disease is modified by medical treatment, and indeed, some patients complain that wearing the collar at night when vision is impaired makes them feel more unsteady (Wyke, 1979). Where there is cervical myelopathy which is progressively deteriorating over a few weeks or months, operation is indicated, regardless of age.

FALLS

Falls are a major problem for elderly persons. Not only is there the risk of serious injury but there is also fear of being unable to get up off the floor afterwards; fear of falling unexpectedly and embarrassingly in a public place, and fear of becoming helpless and dependent. Thus it is not surprising to find that a person with recurrent falls is reluctant to go out of doors and eventually becomes housebound, even bedbound, immobile, demoralized and dependent upon the support of costly social services.

TABLE 2
FEATURES OF FALLS IN THE ELDERLY

1. More common in women than men.

2. Incidence increases linearly with age, although there is a slight fall in incidence among very elderly men.

3. Occur most frequently indoors, especially in the living room and on stairs.

4. Often happen when moving from bed, wheelchair or lavatory.

5. Are particularly common among the socially isolated and those who are depressed or demented.

85

The size of the problem is larger than was once thought. An average district general hospital (serving a population of about 200 000) will have 16 beds continuously occupied by elderly persons admitted because of a fall, yet the number who injure themselves in a fall and need treatment is very small – less than 2% of all those who fall. Population surveys show that about 40% of women and 20% of men over the age of 65 give a history of falls. Thus there is a large amount of disability in the community which is not revealed by accident statistics.

A few points can be summarized here; for a full review see Overstall (1978).

Aetiology

With increasing age postural control declines. Proprioceptive information is only slightly reduced by changes in joints, muscle spindles and peripheral nerves. What is more important is that as a result of degeneration of the cerebellum and its connections the central processes that perceive and integrate proprioceptive signals are critically slowed. Thus reaction times are increased and an elderly person who stumbles, unlike a young one, finds that the speed of his postural reflexes is too slow to prevent a fall. This is the underlying physiological change, but there are a host of additional factors. The two that are most important are general health and mobility. The elderly person who retains his good health, vitality and ability to walk is rarely troubled by falls.

Accidental falls

These account for between one-third and one-half of all falls in the elderly. However the proportion of falls due to this cause declines with increasing age and reflects the greater mobility of the younger group compared with the incapacity of the older who fall for other reasons, such as giddiness.

The majority of accidental falls can be blamed, in part at least, on an unsafe environment: loose carpets, trailing wires, stairs that are too dark, too steep or without an adequate handrail.

Drop attacks

These are sudden falls without warning, where there is no loss of consciousness and no neurological sequelae. They are almost entirely confined to women, and may begin in middle age. Because the attacks are so unexpected and unnerving it is usual for the patient to become very apprehensive and afraid even of walking alone.

The aetiology is not yet entirely clear. Undoubtedly a small proportion of patients have vertebrobasilar insufficiency, but this is not an adequate explanation for the majority who have what is essentially a benign disease that may recur on and off for many years. Recently it has been shown (Hazell, 1979) that most patients, when adequately tested, have a disorder either of the labyrinth or of its central connections. In these patients drop attacks may be precipitated by head movements.

Postural hypotension

This is an important cause of dizziness and falls. The association between falls and rising from bed or a chair must be sought in the history, and the blood pressure measured in the lying and standing positions. The main point is that although postural hypotension is a part of normal ageing (see Chapter 5) it is aggravated by drugs such as diuretics, L-dopa, barbiturates, phenothiazines, tricyclic antidepressants and, of course, antihypertensive agents. These drugs should, if possible, be stopped and the patient mobilized.

Giddiness

This is commonly blamed for falls among the very old. The causes are many but in practice one considers postural hypotension, anxiety neurosis, over-sedation with tranquillizers or hypnotics, cardiac arrhythmias, transient ischaemic attacks, cervical spondylosis and disorders of the labyrinth or cerebellum.

Cardiac arrhythmias

Perhaps the most common cardiac cause of falls is bradycardia due to over-treatment with digoxin or beta-adrenergic blocking drugs. Very brief episodes of cardiac syncope may not actually produce loss of consciousness but are enough to cause a sense of light-headedness and loss of balance. Abrupt changes of rhythm or a run of three or four ectopic beats may be sufficient reason to produce recurrent falls that can be very difficult to diagnose without the aid of 24 hour ambulatory electrocardiographic monitoring (see Chapter 6).

Local causes

Arthritis with limitation of movement of hip, knee or dorsolumbar joints is significantly related to falls. Local muscle weakness may be found in osteomalacia, diabetes, myxoedema and hyperthyroidism.

Drugs

A patient who is sedated at night with a long-acting hypnotic such as a barbiturate or benzodiazepine is at risk of falling both during the night, when he gets up to visit the lavatory, and well into the following morning. The hangover effect of these drugs is well known and they should be avoided in the elderly.

Alcohol and tranquillizers can also blunt the patient's postural control. A long-acting drug such as chlorpropamide may be responsible for early-morning hypoglycaemia and falls.

Premonitory falls

These are falls which precede a sudden and often fatal illness such as a chest infection, stroke, gastrointestinal haemorrhage or myocardial infarct. In most elderly persons the control of postural balance is a delicate one and easily upset by illness. Thus a fall is often a useful warning of a threatened decline in general health.

Management

The first point is to investigate adequately the cause of the falls and to make a diagnosis. Specific problems, such as postural hypotension, are then treated. When vertebrobasilar insufficiency has been shown to be the cause of drop attacks which are related to movements of the head the patient should be given a trial with a cervical collar (see page 85. For labyrinthine disorders there is at present no satisfactory treatment, although labyrinthine sedatives, such as cinnarazine 15 mg three times daily, sometimes help. Even if no precise reason is found for the falls much can still be done. General health can be assessed: anaemia corrected, heart failure treated, painful bunions attended to so as to allow the wearing of proper fitting shoes, etc.

Either as an inpatient, or through the day hospital, the patient is then mobilized. The physiotherapist provides a walking frame, instructs on muscle-strengthening, joint-freeing exercises and gradually builds up the patient's confidence. All the staff have the single aim of encouraging the patient to be safely mobile. Exercises where the patient is taught how to get up from the floor, are helpful. Finally, before discharge the patient's home is visited by the occupational therapist and made as safe as possible.

BLINDNESS

Approximately 69 000 of the population over the age of 65 in the United Kingdom are registered as blind, but many more have less serious degrees of visual impairment. In the survey of the elderly population by Sheldon (1948) only about 6% of individuals had sight sufficiently good to allow them to read without the use of spectacles. The changes which occur in the eye with advancing years lead to a gradual loss of functional efficiency.

Age-changes in the eye

The pupils become small, probably due to increasing rigidity of the iris. Visual acuity is reduced and the visual fields are contracted. The range of accommodation of the lens is limited and it is unable to adapt its shape for the focusing of near objects. At the same time the size of the lens increases and the larger lens is responsible for the development of angle-closure glaucoma. The nucleus of the lens hardens and becomes relatively opaque (nuclear sclerosis) and this is one of the factors favouring the formation of cataract. Intra-ocular pressure increases with advancing age, and this is associated with an increase in prevalence of open-angle glaucoma. In some of these processes it is difficult to distinguish between physiological ageing and pathological conditions.

Presbyobia

The reduction of elasticity of the lens with ageing leads to a gradual limitation in the power of accommodation. Relaxation of the suspensory ligament by the action of the ciliary muscle limits the increase in the anterior–posterior diameter of the lens required for the focusing of near objects. By the age of 45–50 years the lens becomes set in a flat unaccommodated position. Thus the effects of presbyobia become manifest when the near-point of the focus of the lens has receded to an extent which makes reading difficult. This occurs late in initially myopic, and earlier in hypermetropic, individuals. Thus by the age of 50 spectacles are often required for reading and close work, and with further diminution in the power of accommodation in old age a progressive increase in the strength of the near correction is needed.

Cataract

Cataract is present to a disabling degree in 5% of the elderly population. It is rare before the age of 50 except in diabetic subjects who may develop cataract in middle age rather than old age. The lens of the eye is unique in that new lens fibres are constantly being formed throughout life and the old fibres come to lie deeper and more distant from the lens capsule. Ageing in the fibres is accompanied by a reduction in metabolic activity. Opacities, characteristic of cataract, are due to coagulative necrosis in the lens fibres; they may start in the periphery with a typical wedge-shape or as a nuclear cataract in the centre of the lens. The first complaint of the patient may be of a 'speck' before the eye which remains in the same position or of general mistiness of vision. On account of irregular refraction distressing dazzling in bright light occurs. Sometimes the patient maintains that he can see better in the diminished light of the evening when there is pupillary dilatation. As the opacities increase visual acuity becomes progressively impaired. Cataract removal should be considered when the deterioration in vision is sufficient to restrict the patient in his normal activities; it need not wait until the cataract is 'mature'. Confusional states often follow cataract operation and the patient should be informed that with the provision of spectacles to correct the aphakic condition the spherical aberration will lead to distorted vision.

Glaucoma

Patients with both angle-closure glaucoma and open-angle glaucoma usually present to the ophthalmologist when prolonged asymptomatic elevation of intra-ocular pressure has produced pathological cupping of the optic disc and visual field defects due to scotomata. In angle-closure glaucoma the presentation may be acute due to the iris blocking the narrowed filtration angle of the anterior chamber. The sudden marked rise in intra-ocular pressure causes acute pain in the eyes often associated with vomiting, and oedema of the cornea leads to blurring of vision. The pupil becomes dilated and unresponsive to light. This type of severe acute attack is often preceded by milder self-limiting attacks presenting with aching in the eyes, blurring of vision and haloes round lights. Emergency treatment by the ophthalmologist is required for the acute attack using intensive therapy with 2% guttae pilocarpine, followed by intramuscular injection of acetazolamide (500 mg) to suppress aqueous formation. A drainage operation or iridectomy is required to relieve the raised intra-ocular pressure.

In open-angle glaucoma the pressure within the eye rises gradually, due probably to an abnormally high resistance to the outflow of aqueous from the eye. A high incidence of myopia is found in this condition and the large eyeball may be unduly susceptible to raised intra-ocular pressure. The patient often only seeks medical attention when a visual field defect begins to threaten central vision. The aim of treatment is to prevent further deterioration in the visual fields by the control of intra-ocular pressure either medically (e.g. guttae pilocarpine) or by a drainage operation (e.g. anterior sclerectomy).

91

Macular degeneration

This is an important cause of failing vision in old people. The patient often complains that although he is aware of his general surroundings and is able to manage about the house he has difficulty in distinguishing fine detail and is unable to recognize clearly pictures on the television. The degeneration in the retina, which is particularly marked in the region of the macula, is associated with the formation of new vessels within the splits between the membrane layers. The condition may be recognized ophthalmoscopically by the fine pigmentary stippling around the macula, but even with these apparently slight changes the deterioration in vision is usually marked. In the advanced stage the pigment becomes heaped up, and together with the surrounding white areas of choroidal atrophy, a 'moth-eaten' appearance is produced. If the condition can be recognized in a pre-symptomatic stage the use of photocoagulation may prevent progression of the early lesions; this is usually only possible when deterioration in vision has already occurred in one eye but the close follow-up and early treatment of the disease in the other eye enables useful vision to be retained.

Sudden loss of vision

Cataract, glaucoma and macular degeneration are the three disorders most often responsible for the slow deterioration of vision. The much less common sudden loss of vision may be due to occlusion of the central artery of the retina (as the result of thrombosis or micro-emboli); retinal venous occlusion (often in patients with polycythaemia or macroglobulinaemia); retinal detachment; giant-cell arteritis involving the ophthalmic artery, and cortical blindness occurring with bilateral lesions of the visual cortex or as the result of hemianopia on the opposite side in a patient with existing hemianopia. The early detection of giant-cell arteritis and its treatment with corticosteroids are essential to prevent the disaster of ophthalmic artery involvement.

Four per cent of the population suffer from hearing impairment, and three-quarters of the sufferers are over the age of 65. Surveys of the elderly population (for example Sheldon, 1948) show a rising incidence of deafness in old age and after the age of 85 more than 60% have hearing impairment. For the most part the recording of deafness in population surveys is based on the individual's own assessment of his hearing or of the observer's impression of the subject's ability to hear. The findings from different studies show discrepancies but one-third of people over 65 have hearing impairment to produce a social handicap. The few objective studies using audiometry indicate that this may be an underestimate: certainly a high proportion of old people who admit to hearing impairment have not had their hearing assessed.

There are two main forms of deafness:

(1) *Sensori-neural*, which in old age is most often due to presbyacusis; and
(2) *Conductive* due to obstruction by hard wax or to infection in the outer or middle ear.

Many elderly people have mixed deafness due to a degree of both sensori-neural and conductive hearing loss. Other less common causes of deafness to be considered because they occur more often in old age are Paget's disease and the use of drugs (e.g. streptomycin, neomycin and kanomycin) which cause permanent damage to the eighth cranial nerve.

Presbyacusis

This condition is taken to refer to all the changes in the auditory system that are associated with the ageing process as opposed to directly pathological processes. It is, of course, difficult in the older age groups to define what is 'audiologically normal' since not only are there many conditions in old age which affect hearing but throughout

93

life acuity of hearing has been influenced by environmental factors. Population studies using pure-tone audiometry show clearly that hearing loss affecting first of all the higher frequencies increases from the age of 30 onwards (Hinchcliffe, 1959). Sensitivity to pure tones is first impaired at frequencies above 4000 Hz, but with each successive decade in adult life progressive impairment occurs and by the age of 60 it is apparent at frequencies above 1000 Hz. It is likely that the degenerative changes throughout the auditory system including the brain account for the functional abnormalities in presbyacusis. The salient features are shown in Table 3.

TABLE 3
CHARACTERISTICS OF PRESBYACUSIS

Impairment of	*Effect*
1. Auditory threshold sensitivity	hearing loss for higher tones first
2. Frequency discrimination	difficulty in distinguishing tones of different frequencies
3. Temporal discrimination	distortion of time-relationships and delay in central processing
4. Localization of sound	difficulty in ascertaining direction of sound
5. Loudness perception (hypersensitivity)	recruitment – narrowing of gap between sounds being inaudible and hearing too loud for comfort
6. Phoneme discrimination	decrease in intelligibility of speech

Tinnitus and vertigo are commonly associated with presbyacusis but neither symptom is related to the severity of hearing loss. Although pure tone audiometry is the most widely used procedure for the assessment of hearing, it has its limitations. Many patients with presbyacusis have disproportionately greater difficulties in speech discrimination than one would expect from the results of the pure tone audiogram. The various components of speech have different dur-

94

ations; consonants have a shorter duration than vowels and as they are mainly in the higher range of frequencies phoneme discrimination is poorer for consonants than it is for vowels. Moreover much of the information in speech is encoded in the consonant sounds and when these cannot be well identified speech becomes unintelligible.

Stevenson (1975) has investigated these aspects of presbyacusis by the use of an automated speech audiometry test system. Errors in phoneme discrimination can be represented pictorially in a directed graph form (digraph). The general directedness of the identification errors in the digraph is away from the fricatives and front articulated consonants. Thus consonants which are difficult to lip-read on account of their articulation position (/K/ /G/ etc). are least susceptible to acoustic misidentification, while that set which is easy to lip-read is most liable to acoustic misidentification. This emphasizes the importance of lip-reading for the elderly individual with presbyacusis.

Mental and social consequences
Hearing impairment has a considerable effect on the lives of old people. When severe it is a form of sensory deprivation which leads to social isolation; social isolation is in turn associated with many other unmet needs in the elderly. Sometimes the handicap in communication is so great that the mental state of the patient becomes impaired and he develops an acute or chronic confusional state (Hodkinson, 1973). There is also an association between deafness and paranoid psychosis. Patients with paranoid psychosis have more severe hearing loss than those in the general population of similar age. The hearing loss is usually of long standing, and as there is often a long interval between the onset of deafness and the onset of psychosis it would seem that the correction of hearing impairment by hearing aids might be of value in preventing mental deterioration.

Management
The first problem is that of ascertainment. Elderly population surveys show that at least one-third of those who complain of deafness have not had any measurement of their hearing impairment. Hearing testing should include speech audiometry since pure tone audiometry

95

alone will not reveal the extent of the hearing difficulties caused by impaired speech discrimination. Most tests of hearing are carried out under acoustically ideal conditions which bear little relation to normal situations; the effects of background noise on speech intelligibility should also be assessed.

The most satisfactory means of improving communication is by means of amplification with a hearing aid. The frequency range of the amplifier should extend to 4 kHz and above with selective amplification at the higher frequencies. Nevertheless there are still limitations; the recruitment phenomenon leads to intolerable hypersensitivity to high-intensity sounds and impaired phoneme discrimination for consonant sounds of short duration remains imperfect with consequent poor speech intelligibility. Some of these problems might be overcome by incorporating an automatic volume control or peak clipping.

Hearing aids worn at ear level have some advantages over body-worn aids. The aid can be turned towards the sound source by movement of the head, there is no noise from the rubbing of clothes and psychologically this type of aid is more acceptable. Binaural aids improve the discrimination of speech in background noise, and this leads to better speech intelligibility; they also improve localization of sound.

Although there has been a considerable increase in the provision of aids for the elderly deaf during the last 30 years, still an unacceptably high proportion of old people with aids fail to use them. The effective use of hearing aids depends on the availability of good maintenance and advisory facilities with very careful follow-up supervision of those provided with aids; advice and education must also be directed towards relatives, friends and those who care for the elderly professionally.

Hearing aids with their limitations should be regarded as an adjuvant to good communication. When talking to the elderly deaf person encouragement should be given to lip-reading by allowing light to fall on the speaker's mouth; the voice should be moderately loud and not shouting, and speech should be at a slower speed to take account of the delay in comprehension of speech by the higher centres.

96

REFERENCES

Blackwood, W., Hallpike, J. F., Kocen, R. S. and Mair, W. G. P. (1969). Atheromatous disease of the carotid arterial system and embolism from the heart in cerebral infarction: a morbid anatomical study. *Brain*, **92,** 897

Brain, Lord (1963). Some unsolved problems of cervical spondylosis. *Br. Med. J.*, **1,** 771

Canadian Cooperative Study Group (1978). A randomized trial of aspirin and sulfinpyrazone in threatened stroke. *N. Engl. J. Med.*, **299,** 53

Critchley, M. (1931). The neurology of old age. *Lancet*, **i,** 1119

Fisher, C. M. (1954). Occlusion of the carotid arteries. *Arch. Neurol. Psychiat.*, **72,** 187

Hakim, A. M. and Mathieson, G. (1978). Basis of dementia in Parkinson's disease. *Lancet*, **ii,** 729

Harris, A. I., Cox, E. and Smith, C. R. W. (1971). *The Handicapped and Impaired in Great Britain*. Part 1. Office of Population Censuses and Surveys. (London: HMSO)

Hazell, J. W. P. (1979). Vestibular problems of balance. *Age and Ageing* (In press)

Hinchcliffe, R. (1959). The threshold of hearing as a function of age. *Acoustica*, **9,** 303

Hodkinson, H. M. (1973). Mental impairment in the elderly. *J. R. Coll. Physicians, London*, **7,** 305

Hunt, L. B. (1973). The elderly in hospital: recent trends in use of medical resources. *Br. Med. J.* (Suppl.), Dec. 22nd, p. 83

Hutchinson, E. C. and Yates, P. O. (1957). Caroticovertebral stenosis. *Lancet*, **i,** 2

Lees, A. J., Shaw, K. M., Kohout, L. J., Elseworth, J. D., Sandler, M. and Youdhim, M. B. H. (1977). Deprenyl in Parkinson's disease. *Lancet*, **ii,** 791

Llarsson, O., Marinovich, N. and Barber, K. (1976). Double blind study of glycerol therapy in early stroke. *Lancet*, **i,** 832

Marquardsen, J. (1969). The natural history of acute cerebrovascular disease. *Acta. Neurol. Scand.*, **45** (Suppl.), 38

Mulley, G., and Arie, T. (1978). Treating stroke: home or hospital? *Br. Med. J.*, **2,** 1321

Mulley, G., Wilcox, R. G. and Mitchell, J. R. A. (1978). Dexamethasone in acute stroke. *Br. Med. J.*, **2,** 994

Oxbury, J. M., Greenhall, R. C. D. and Grainger, K. M. R. (1975). Predicting the outcome of stroke: acute stage after cerebral infarction. *Br. Med. J.*, **3,** 125

Overstall, P. W. (1978). Falls in the elderly – epidemiology, aetiology, and management. In B. Isaacs (ed.). *Recent Advances in Geriatric Medicine.* (Edinburgh: Churchill Livingstone)

Sheldon, J. H. (1948). *The Social Medicine of Old Age.* (London: Oxford University Press)

Schen, R. J. and Benaroya, Y. (1976). Hypoglycaemic coma due to chlorpropamide. *Age and Ageing,* **5,** 31

Stevenson, P. W. (1975). Responses to speech audiometry and phonemic discrimination patterns in the elderly. *Audiology,* **14,** 185

Storey, G. O. (1971). Medical treatment. In M. Wilkinson (ed.). *Cervical Spondylosis.* (London: Heinemann)

Thompson, P. L. and Robinson, J. S. (1978). Stroke after acute myocardial infarction: relation to infarct size. *Br. Med. J.*, **2,** 457

Wyke, B. (1979). Cervical articular contributions to posture and gait: their relation to senile disequilibrium. *Age and Ageing* (In press)

5
Autonomic nervous system

Disorder of autonomic function is often concerned in the causation of two common clinical conditions in old age – postural hypotension and hypothermia. It may also be a factor in the development of heat illness, disturbances of oesophageal and gastrointestinal motility and in some cases of urinary retention and incontinence (see Chapter 11).

AGE-CHANGES IN AUTONOMIC FUNCTION

Investigations based on examination of the elderly population living at home indicate that impairment of autonomic function is common in old age. Caird and his colleagues (1973) found that the incidence of postural hypotension increased with age; thus a fall of 20 mmHg or more in systolic pressure was observed in 16% of those aged 65–74 years and in 30% of those aged 75 and over. They believe that autonomic dysfunction is the underlying cause and this commonly interacts with other factors to produce postural hypotension in old age (see Table 2). In the elderly individual it is often difficult to determine the relative importance of these two components.

Autonomic dysfunction leading to postural hypotension may be due to impairment of the afferent part of the baroreceptor reflex arc, to

99

lesions in the central structures, or to impairment of function in the effector system which is responsible for systemic arteriolar constriction and possibly constriction of venous reservoirs. In addition it is likely that failure to control the splanchnic vascular bed plays an important part in the development of postural hypotension.

Thermoregulatory function has also been investigated in the elderly population. Fox and his colleagues (1973) measured the body temperatures in a random sample of 1020 people over the age of 65 living at home in Great Britain during the first three months of 1972. Lowering of deep body temperature (as measured by urine temperature) was significantly correlated with advancing age. In 10% of subjects the deep body temperature was less than 35.5 °C and these individuals were thought to have some degree of thermoregulatory failure, as shown by an inability to maintain an adequate core–periphery temperature gradient. The mean difference between the urine temperature and the hand temperature in this group was 2.9 °C compared with 4.6 °C for those in the 'normal' temperature group whose deep body temperatures were 36.0 °C and above. This was confirmed when a 15% subsample of the participants in the Camden survey were submitted to thermoregulatory function tests involving the measurement of physiological responses to a cycle of neutral, cool and warm environments created by a specially designed air conditioned test bed.

It was found that shivering occurred during the cooling period in 12% of the elderly subjects as compared with 30% in a group of young adults. Sweating occurred in all the young subjects but in only about half the elderly during the period of warming. Abnormal peripheral blood flow patterns on cooling and warming (see Figure 1, curves B and C) were found in 56% of the men and 45% of the women; these were found to be rare in the young control subjects.

When tests of thermoregulatory function were repeated 4 years later in 43 of the subjects a significantly higher proportion had low resting peripheral blood flow (less than 5 ml/100 ml hand tissue per minute) and a higher proportion had a non-constrictor response on cooling (Collins *et al.*, 1977). In the group with a normal peripheral blood flow pattern it was found that there was a significant increase in deep body temperature required to initiate sweating on warming,

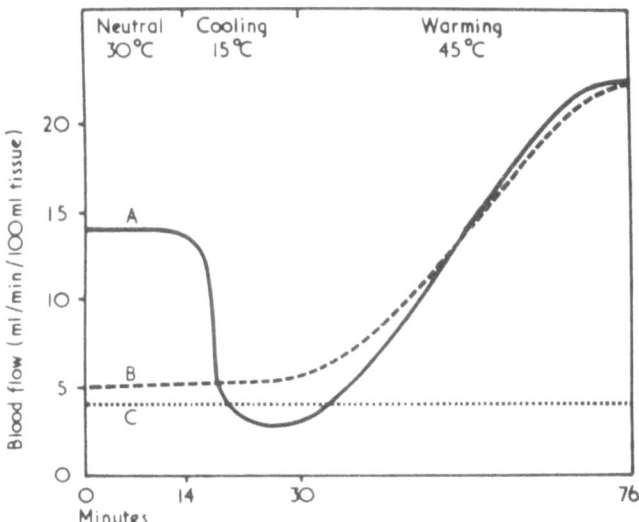

Figure 1   Blood flow responses of (A) normal people; (B) non-constrictors; and (C) non-constrictor/non-dilators

compared with the level in the first study. Thus these physiological studies have established, both on a cross-sectional and longitudinal basis, that there is an age-related decline in autonomic function which leads to impairment of thermoregulatory capacity in a high proportion of old people.

PATHOLOGICAL CONDITIONS AFFECTING AUTONOMIC FUNCTION

A number of pathological processes and drugs may lead to dysfunction in the autonomic nervous system. These are summarized in Table 1.

Shy-Drager syndrome

Although this is a rare disease it is mentioned first since all the manifestations for autonomic failure are to be found in the clinical picture.

101

TABLE 1

PATHOLOGICAL CONDITIONS AFFECTING AUTONOMIC FUNCTION

Central disturbances	*Autonomic neuropathy*
Shy-Drager syndrome	Diabetes mellitus
Parkinsonism	Malignancy
	(especially bronchus and pancreas)
Wernicke's encephalopathy	
Cerebrovascular disease	Amyloidosis
Tabes dorsalis	Acute infective polyneuropathy
Paraplegia	Vitamin B complex deficiency
Chronic alcoholism	Chronic alcoholism
Psychotropic drugs	Drugs

Shy and Drager (1960) described two cases of a neurological syndrome associated with orthostatic hypotension, defective sweating and sphincter disturbances, to be followed by the appearance of somatic neurological manifestations. The fall in systolic blood pressure on standing often exceeds 50 mmHg and the postural symptoms include dizziness, faintness, ataxia and headache. The somatic manifestations, which may appear after an interval of 6 months to 20 years, include unsteadiness of gait, rigidity of the limbs, tremor and other features of Parkinsonism. Occasionally the somatic disorders precede the dysautonomia and when these take the form of Parkinsonism an erroneous diagnosis of paralysis agitans may be made.

Parkinsonism

In the majority of cases the characteristic clinical features of Parkinsonism are present (see Chapter 4) and the autonomic disturbances are recognized later. Investigation of autonomic function shows a resting blood pressure lower than expected for the patient's age and sex, orthostatic hypotension and increased sensitivity to noradrenaline, impairment of thermoregulatory function with patchy loss of sweating, and abnormal bladder function. L-dopa therapy of patients with uncomplicated Parkinsonism sometimes first reveals evidence of autonomic dysfunction, and it is possible that autonomic disturbances in paralysis agitans occur more frequently than generally recognized.

Wernicke's encephalopathy

This condition is due to thiamine deficiency often associated with alcoholism (see Chapter 10) and the characteristic petechial haemorrhages are to be found in the walls of the third ventricle, the hypothalamus and mamillary bodies. Birchfield (1964) found postural hypotension in 32 of a series of 40 cases. Other clinical features include ophthalmoplegia (26), nystagmus (32), ataxia (in all of the 25 cases tested) peripheral neuropathy (29) and Korsakoff's psychosis (28). Hypothermia can also occur, and Phillip and Smith (1973) state that the disorder of temperature regulation is often overlooked in most cases of Wernicke's encephalopathy.

Cerebrovascular disease

Postural hypotension is common in elderly inpatients and it is observed more frequently than in old people at home. It has been attributed to cerebrovascular disease, but associated factors are age and debility. Postural hypotension and impairment of temperature regulation may also be due to psychotropic drugs, especially the phenothiazines, which are commonly prescribed in patients with cerebrovascular disease.

Autonomic neuropathy

Diabetes mellitus is the commonest cause of autonomic neuropathy associated with peripheral neuropathy. Other less frequent causes are shown in Table 1. In diabetes the symptoms include impotence, dizziness and faintness due to postural hypotension, intermittent nocturnal diarrhoea, intermittent vomiting, gastric fullness, dysuria,

103

reduced sweating in the legs and impairment of temperature regulation leading to hypothermia. The incidence of peripheral neuropathy as a complication of diabetes is uncertain and the frequency reported in the literature varies from 4 to 93%. It is even more difficult to estimate the frequency of autonomic neuropathy, but when autonomic function tests are carried out it is found in 25–75% of patients with diabetic peripheral neuropathy. Ewing and his colleagues (1976) emphasize that it has a bad prognosis; the mortality in $2\frac{1}{2}$ years in a series of diabetic patients was twice as great when autonomic neuropathy was present compared with those in which tests of autonomic function were normal.

CLINICAL SYNDROMES

I. Postural hypotension

Aetiology
The principal factors responsible for postural hypotension in the elderly are summarized in Table 2.

TABLE 2
CAUSES OF POSTURAL HYPOTENSION

1. Physiological decline in autonomic function due to ageing with or without one or more of the following: absent ankle jerks, varicose veins, drugs, anaemia, bacteriuria, hyponatraemia

2. Drugs affecting autonomic function, especially phenothiazine tranquillizers and hypotensive agents

3. Diseases involving the autonomic nervous system (see Table 1)

Clinical features
In many instances postural hypotension is asymptomatic; the autoregulation of the cerebral circulation is able to compensate for the fall in systemic arterial pressure. In other cases when autoregulation fails, possibly as a result of cerebrovascular disease, or if the

104

postural fall in blood pressure is excessive the patient complains of weakness, faintness, dizziness, loss of balance or blacking out of vision, especially when rising from the lying position. Falls associated with postural hypotension may lead to fractures and to accidental hypothermia when the old person is living in cold rooms. Whenever postural hypotension is discovered a search should be made for somatic neurological involvement including peripheral neuropathy, olivo-ponto-cerebellar degeneration, pyramidal tract lesions and Parkinsonism. Even in the absence of clinical signs of multiple system degeneration elsewhere in the nervous system it is possible that deterioration in autonomic function is associated with a physiological decline in somatic function. Thus Overstall and his colleagues (1977 and 1978) have shown that body sway is greater in those old people with postural hypotension compared with age-matched controls, and this increased sway is unrelated to the level of blood pressure.

Management

Appropriate treatment should be given to those patients who are found to have correctable causes of postural hypotension. The use of sympathomimetic drugs has proved disappointing. The administration of fludrocortisone is more promising; it expands blood volume so that even when pooling occurs in the dependent capacity vessels there is sufficient blood to maintain venous return to the heart. The dose given must be large (0.5–2.0 mg per day) and in the elderly there is danger of precipitating congestive cardiac failure or pulmonary oedema. Pooling of blood on assuming the upright position may also be prevented by mechanical means such as the wearing of anti-G trousers designed primarily for airmen. Although successful this is not usually a very practical measure in the elderly. To be effective elastic stockings have to be full length and used in combination with an elastic abdominal support.

Lang and others (1975) have reported significant improvement in postural hypotension treated with dihydroergotamine (2 mg three times a day). The effects of dihydroergotamine may be due largely to its powerful and relatively selective action on the capacity vessels in the peripheral circulation. Recently, Perkins and Lee (1978) have shown that severe postural hypotension may respond to therapy with the prostaglandin-synthetase inhibitor, flurbiprofen (50 mg twice daily) combined with fludrocortisone. The patient they describe was able to lead a normal life after 3 months combined therapy, whereas prior to treatment she was unable to stand owing to syncope associated with a fall in blood pressure to a level which was unrecordable.

II. Accidental hypothermia

Hypothermia is defined as a state of subnormal body temperature in which the deep body temperature falls below 35 °C (95 °F). It became recognized in Great Britain during the 1960s as a problem particularly affecting old people. The term accidental hypothermia is used to imply that the lowering of deep body temperature is unintentional, and it has to be distinguished from hypothermia which is induced therapeutically.

Incidence

Even up to 15 years ago accidental hypothermia in the elderly was thought to be a rare condition. It was known to occur in association with certain diseases, for example, myxoedema, hypopituitarism and alcoholism. The British Medical Association's Committee on accidental hypothermia in the elderly (1964), after reviewing descriptions of cases reported in the literature, concluded that there was no accurate information on the prevalence of the condition. The hospital reports indicated that very few cases were recognized clinically before admission and elderly people with hypothermia suffered a high mortality.

Duguid, Simpson and Stowers (1961) described 23 cases occurring in Scotland; all the patients were elderly and developed hypothermia indoors. The deep body temperatures on admission, as measured by a rectal thermometer, ranged from 22.8 °C to 31.9 °C and only seven (30%) of the patients survived. Rosin and Exton-Smith (1964) described 32 patients with hypothermia, half of whom were seen during the very cold winter of 1962/63. With the exception of one aged 39

106

years their ages ranged from 60 to 92 years. Although ten patients were found lying on the floor, the others suffered from lesser degrees of exposure – ten were in bed at home, two were sitting in a chair and one developed hypothermia in hospital. The results of a Royal College of Physicians survey (1966) in ten hospital groups during the months February, March and April 1965 showed an incidence of hypothermia in 0.68% of all patients admitted, of whom 42% were over the age of 65. This indicated that about 3800 elderly patients were admitted with hypothermia to hospitals in Great Britain during these three winter months. Ten years later, a second Royal College of Physicians survey conducted at two London Hospitals in January to April 1975 showed that 3.6% of patients over the age of 65 admitted to hospital were hypothermic, a prevalence considerably higher than that of the previous College study (Goldman *et al.*, 1977).

Aetiology
Usually multiple factors are involved in the aetiology of accidental hypothermia in old people, and the more important are shown in Table 3.

TABLE 3
CAUSES OF ACCIDENTAL HYPOTHERMIA IN THE ELDERLY

---

1. *Exogenous* – cold exposure
   (75–90°$_{0}$ of cases, indoors)
2. *Endogenous*
   - (a) *Physiological* (i) Impaired thermoregulation
     - (ii) Impaired temperature discrimination
   - (b) *Pathological* (i) Endocrine: myxoedema, hypopituitarism, diabetes
     - (ii) Neurological: hemiplegia, Parkinsonism
     - (iii) Locomotor: arthritis
     - (iv) Mental: Confusional states, dementia
     - (v) Infections: bronchopneumonia
     - (vi) Circulatory: cardiac infarction, pulmonary embolism
     - (vii) Drugs: phenothiazines, antidepressants, alcohol

Exogenous factors   Exposure to cold is an over-riding cause and the Royal College of Physicians survey (1966) showed a clear relationship between the incidence of hypothermia and a low environmental temperature. The number of cases rose considerably when the ambient temperature fell below 0 °C. A common story is of an old person who falls after attempting to get out of bed at night; he remains on the floor for several hours, often partly clad, and is discovered the next day by a neighbour or a home-help. Thus the exposure is likely to be longer when the old person lives alone and is socially isolated. Many cases, however, occur when the old person is in bed at night apparently well-covered with clothes. In these instances insufficient body heat is being generated, so that even good external insulation is ineffective.

Endogenous factors   The high prevalence of accidental hypothermia in old people can mainly be accounted for by the physiological decline in thermoregulatory function which has been clearly revealed in both cross-sectional and longitudinal studies (see page 100). In addition many old people have a diminished sensitivity to cold. Tests of digital thermo-sensation (Collins *et al.*, 1977) show that young people can perceive mean temperature differences of about 0.8 °C whereas elderly subjects could discriminate only between mean temperature differences of 2.5 °C and some are unable to perceive differences of 5 °C or more. It is likely that a lessened sensitivity to cold is one of the reasons for the relatively large numbers of old people who appear to be able to tolerate cold conditions without discomfort. Nevertheless, such individuals may be at risk of over-taxing the heat-conserving capacity of a failing thermoregulatory system.

Although some old people admitted to hospital suffer from primary accidental hypothermia (that is, the hypothermia is the result of cold exposure and failing thermoregulation), in the majority pathological conditions are present. A stroke may be responsible for the initial fall, and cold exposure because the patient remains immobile on the floor. In a number of neurological and locomotor disorders immobility is a factor limiting the amount of heat generated, and in Parkinsonism there may be an additional factor of autonomic dysfunction. Patients with confusional states and dementia may be unaware of environmental hazards and there is some evidence for impairment of temperature regulation in dementia. The psychotropic drugs prescribed for these conditions may also affect thermoregulation. Bronchopneumonia may precipitate hypothermia and it usually develops insidiously in those suffering from hypothermia due to other causes. Other severe infections, cardiac infarction and pulmonary embolism can cause an acute derangement of thermoregulatory mechanisms.

Clinical features
Descriptions of the clinical features are given in the reports of cases treated in hospital by Duguid and her colleagues (1961) and by Rosin and Exton-Smith (1964).

Appearance   The patient usually has a grey appearance due to a mixture of pallor and cyanosis. The skin is cold to touch, not only in exposed parts of the body but also in those parts normally covered; for example, the axillae and the abdominal wall. The puffy facial appearance, the slow cerebration and the husky voice may be mistaken for myxoedema.

Level of consciousness   Below 32 °C clouding of consciousness and drowsiness are usually apparent. The lower the body temperature the more likely is the patient to be comatose, and in the series described by Rosin and Exton-Smith (1964) three-quarters of the patients with rectal temperatures below 27 °C were unconscious.

Central nervous system   The reflexes are sluggish and the muscular hypertonus which replaces shivering at low temperatures gives rise to neck stiffness simulating meningism and to rigidity of the abdominal wall. An involuntary flapping tremor of the arms and legs has been observed in some patients (Rosin and Exton-Smith, 1964).

109

Cardiovascular system   The heart rate slows in response to cold, due to sinus bradycardia or slow atrial fibrillation. The electrocardiogram usually shows some degree of heart block, with an increase in PR interval (in patients with sinus rhythm) and there is delay in intraventricular conduction.

A pathogenic sign is the appearance of a 'J' wave (see Figure 2), shown by a characteristic deflection at the junction of the QRS and ST segment, (Osborn, 1953; Emslie-Smith, 1958). The size of these waves varies from patient to patient and they are not related to the severity of the hypothermia; they are often absent altogether. In any one individual the height of the wave diminishes as the patient recovers and the deep body temperature rises. A fall in arterial blood pressure is an ominous sign.

Respiratory system   Respirations are slow and shallow. When the hyponoea is severe a fall in arterial oxygen saturation occurs with consequent anoxia of the tissues which may determine the prognosis. Bronchopneumonia may be present without the usual clinical signs. Basal crepitations may also be due to cold injury to the alveoli.

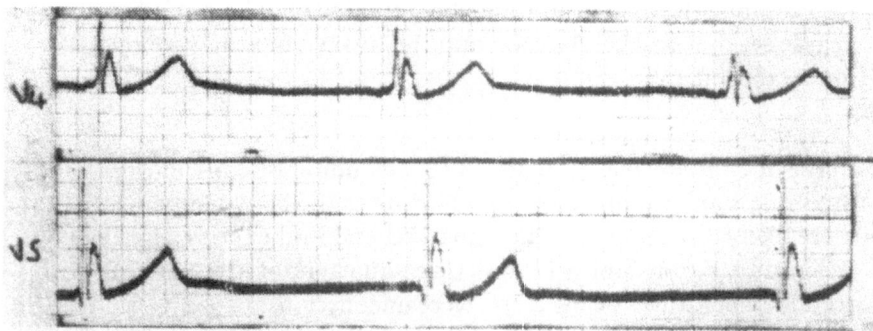

Figure 2   Electrocardiogram showing well marked J waves in V4 and V5 in a man aged 79 who had a rectal temperature of 29°C on admission to hospital.

Alimentary system   Acute pancreatitis is often found at post-mortem examination. A rise in the serum amylase was found in 11 of the 15 cases tested by Duguid *et al.* (1961). Fulminating pancreatitis, a condition generally accompanied by pain and shock, may give rise to few signs in the hypothermic patient. It should be suspected if the patient winces when firm pressure is applied to the epigastrium.

Management
Experience has shown that rapid re-warming of the elderly person suffering from hypothermia is hazardous. If, however, the temperature is allowed to rise slowly and spontaneously the period of hypothermia is greatly prolonged, and when there has already been long exposure at home, irreversible changes in the tissues may take place. In the absence of more satisfactory methods of warming the body core without the application of external heat, one of two therapeutic regimes is advocated.

Mild to moderate hypothermia (32 °C to 35 °C)   The room temperature in a cubicle is maintained at about 27 °C to allow the deep body temperature to rise about 0.5 °C per hour. The patient is barrier nursed and a broad-spectrum antibiotic is administered in an attempt to prevent bronchopneumonia. Oxygen is given if tissue anoxia is present. The pulse and blood pressure must be monitored and if there is a drop in pressure during the course of treatment the patient is cooled again temporarily by lowering the room temperature.

Severe hypothermia (deep body temperature less than 32 °C)   The patient must be treated in an intensive care unit and the additional measures required are: institution of positive pressure ventilation; insertion of a central venous catheter for the measurement of pressure and for the administration of warm fluids; correction of dehydration and acidosis, and the monitoring of deep body temperature either continuously (by a thermistor in the external auditory meatus) or half-hourly (by a rectal thermometer).

Many patients treated with these regimes regain a normal deep body temperature within 12–24 hours, but the later outcome is dependent on the degree and duration of the hypothermia and on the nature and the severity of the causative clinical condition.

111

III. Heat-related illness and heat stroke

It is now recognized that the number of deaths from all causes provides a more valid measure of the effects of extremes of temperature than the numbers revealed by death certification as due to heat illness or hypothermia. The adverse effects of high environmental temperatures are seen mainly in the elderly population, and mortality in the older age groups increases dramatically during heat waves.

Mortality in heat waves
The United States Vital Statistics Reports for the Nation for the years 1957–67 reveal that during heat waves persons over the age of 50 show an increase in deaths from all causes beyond the numbers expected, and progressively so with advancing years (Ellis, 1971). In a study of the causes of deaths which occurred in the heat waves in New York City in July 1972 and in August and September 1973 excess deaths in the aged population were due mainly to ischaemic heart disease and, to a lesser extent, to cerebrovascular disease (Ellis *et al.*, 1975). It was notable that only a small proportion of deaths were certified as due to the effects of heat illness, and none was certified to be due to heat illness alone. In the more moderate climate of England and Wales mortality also changes with fluctuations in environmental temperature (OPCS Monitor, 1975 and 1976). It is lowest when the mean temperature is about 17–18 °C and rises with mean temperature above about 20 °C. Lyster (1976) has pointed out that these variations are obscured when monthly patterns of mortality are studied, but are only revealed by analysis of weekly mortality figures. This is because peak deaths during heat waves are followed by an exceptionally low trough; that is, when a heat wave leads to a sudden increase in mortality of those at greatest risk, fewer die in the immediately succeeding weeks.

Aetiology
Impairment of thermoregulatory function due to diminished or absent sweating is thought to be one of the factors responsible for the occurrence of heat stroke and for the increased mortality in the elderly

112

population during heat waves (Ellis *et al.*, 1976). Phenothiazine drugs, which interfere with thermoregulation and suppress sweating, produce additional hazards for old people in hot weather.

Clinical features of heat stroke in the aged

In the series of 25 fatal cases described by Levine (1969) the average rectal temperature on admission was 41.3 °C. There was a high incidence of chronic disease: 72% had arteriosclerotic heart disease and other common conditions were congestive cardiac failure, diabetes mellitus, Parkinsonism and the effects of recent or old stroke. A history of the prodromal phases was rarely available but some patients complained of weakness, nausea, vomiting, dizziness, headache, breathlessness, anorexia and a feeling of warmth. Important clinical features were dehydration with anhydrosis in the majority of patients (84%), coma with complete unresponsiveness to painful stimuli (72%), and signs of pulmonary consolidation (76%) often due to gram-negative staphylococcal infection. Six of the 15 patients in whom the serum sodium was estimated had levels above 150 mmol/l and eight of 22 patients had serum chloride levels of more than 105 mmol/l. Elderly patients probably differ from younger patients in their ability to combat severe and rapidly developing water dehydration because of depressed sensorium, weakness, and failure of the cardiovascular and renal mechanisms for water conservation. The transfer of adequate quantities of heat from the body core structures to the periphery where heat is lost is dependent upon circulatory adjustments which are deficient in old people with cardiovascular disease.

Management

The reduction of deep body temperature is usually achieved by cold water sponges and iced baths, but the success of rapid external cooling requires vigorous massage to the skin to counteract rapid reflex peripheral vasoconstriction produced by the markedly elevated core to shell thermal gradient induced by external cooling. Circulatory shock occurs in many heat stroke victims, and the administration of steroids in an attempt to overcome this is of doubtful value. Intravenous fluids

113

are required to counteract water and/or salt depletion but there is considerable danger of precipitating pulmonary oedema. The prognosis is very poor due often, as in the case of accidental hypothermia, to the serious nature of the underlying diseases which predispose the elderly to disorders of thermoregulation.

REFERENCES

Birchfield, R. I. (1964). Postural hypotension in Wernicke's disease. *Am. J. Med.*, **36**, 404

British Medical Association Memorandum (1964). Accidental hypothermia in the elderly. *Br. Med. J.*, **2**, 1255

Caird, F. I., Andrews, G. R. and Kennedy, R. D. (1973). Effect of posture on blood pressure in the elderly. *Br. Heart J.*, **35**, 527

Collins, K. J., Dore, C., Exton-Smith, A. N., Fox, R. H., MacDonald, I. C. and Woodward, P. M. (1977). Accidental hypothermia and impaired temperature homeostasis in the elderly. *Br. Med. J.*, **1**, 353

Duguid, H., Simpson, R. G. and Stowers, J. M. (1961). Accidental hypothermia. *Lancet*, **ii**, 1213

Ellis, F. P. (1971). Mortality from heat illness and heat-aggravated illness in the United States. *Environ. Res.*, **5**, 1

Ellis, F. P., Exton-Smith, A. N., Foster, K. G. and Weiner, J. S., (1976). Mortality during heat waves in very young and very old persons and eccrine sweating. *Israel J. Med. Sci.*, **12**, 111

Ellis, F. P., Nelson, F. and Pincus, L. (1975). Mortality during heat waves in New York City, July 1972 and August–September, 1973. *Environ. Res.*, **10**, 1

Emslie-Smith, D. (1958). Accidental hypothermia: a common condition with a pathognomonic ECG. *Lancet*, **ii**, 492

Ewing, D. J., Campbell, I. W. and Clarke, B. F. (1976). Mortality in diabetic autonomic neuropathy. *Lancet*, **i**, 601

Fox, R. H., Woodward, P. M., Exton-Smith, A. N., Green, M. F., Donnison, D. V. and Wicks, M. H. (1973). Body temperatures in the elderly: a national study of physiological, social and environmental conditions. *Br. Med. J.*, **1**, 200

Goldman, A., Exton-Smith, A. N., Francis, G. and O'Brien, A. (1977). A pilot study of low body temperatures in old people admitted to hospital. *J. Roy. Coll. Physicians*, **2**, 291

Lang, E., Jansen, W. and Pfaff, W., (1975). Orthostatische hypotenie bei älteren Menschen. *Med. Klin.*, **70,** 1979

Levine, J. A., (1969). Heat stroke in the aged. *Am. J. Med.*, **47,** 251

Lyster, W. R. (1976). Death in summer. *Lancet*, **ii,** 469

OPCS Monitor, London (1975 and 1976). Office of Population Censuses and Surveys

Osborn, J. J. (1953). Experimental hypothermia: respiratory and blood pH changes in relation to cardiac function. *Am. J. Physiol.*, **175,** 389

Overstall, P. W., Imms, F. J., Exton-Smith, A. N. and Johnston, A. L. (1977). Falls in the elderly related to postural imbalance. *Br. Med. J.*, **1,** 261

Overstall, P. W., Johnson, A. L. and Exton-Smith, A. N. (1978). Instability and falls in the elderly. *Age and Ageing*, **7** (Suppl.), 92

Perkins, C. M. and Lee, M. R. (1978). Flurbiprofen and fludrocortisone in severe autonomic neuropathy, *Lancet*, **ii,** 1058

Phillip, G. and Smith, J. F. (1973). Hypothermia and Wernicke's encephalopathy, *Lancet*, **ii,** 122

Rosin, A. and Exton-Smith, A. N. (1964). Clinical features of accidental hypothermia with observations on thyroid function. *Br. Med. J.*, **1,** 16

Royal College of Physicians of London (1966). Report of Committee on Accidental Hypothermia

Shy, G. M. and Drager, G. A. (1960). A neurological syndrome associated with orthostatic hypotension. *Arch. Neurol.*, **2,** 511

6
Cardiovascular system

Vessels

The effects of ageing on the aorta are: cystic medial fibrosis; elastin fragmentation, characterized by disruption of elastic lamellae; fibrosis, defined as an increase in collagen at the expense of smooth muscle; and medionecrosis. These are probably wear and tear changes secondary to haemodynamic events (Schlatmann and Becker, 1977), and are most marked in the ascending aorta, arch and the lower limb arteries. As a result of smooth muscle atrophy and the increase in collagen, larger arteries tend to elongate and dilate. The intima thickens due to the deposition of collagen between the endothelium and internal elastic lamina.

Superimposed on these changes is the formation of atherosclerosis, which appears to be dependent on various environmental and metabolic factors and not age alone.

Heart

In the myocardium there is atrophy of smooth muscle, an increase in

117

fibrous tissue, an excess of the normal brown pigment ('brown atrophy') and deposition of amyloid. Calcification of the mitral valve ring and the aortic cusps is common and found only in the elderly (Pomerance, 1965). The thickness of the diastolic wall and heart mass increase with age.

Physiology

The changes in the walls of the aorta and large vessels cause a rise in systolic but not in diastolic pressure. Some of the changes in the heart associated with ageing may result from hypertrophy, since there are many similarities between the aged heart and the heart hypertrophied by some pathological high-impedance states (Gerstenblith, Lakatta and Weisfeldt, 1976). In the aged heart at rest the duration of cardiac contraction and relaxation is prolonged, peripheral vascular resistance is increased, cardiac output is lower and impedence to left ventricular ejection is greater. However there are no important changes in the function of the heart as a pump.

Ageing seriously affects the response of the heart to exercise. Maximal heart rate, stroke volume and A-V oxygen difference are all lower. The reasons for this poor, age-related response to stress are not known but are probably due to a decline in myofibrillar ATPase activity.

HEART FAILURE

Age alone is not an acceptable explanation for failure, and old hearts fail for much the same reasons as young ones. In a necropsy study of patients aged over 75 years Pomerance (1965) found that only 2% of those with heart failure had normal hearts. In the failure cases the commonest finding was ischaemic heart disease (48.5%) followed, in order of frequency, by: degenerative calcific changes in mitral ring or aortic cusp, hypertension, senile cardiac amyloidosis, endocarditis, cor pulmonale, calcified aortic stenosis, rheumatic heart disease, mucoid degeneration of the mitral valve and syphilis. The most striking feature of the failure cases was the multiplicity of pathological findings that increased with age.

118

Clinical features

In addition to the pathological causes of heart failure listed above it is usually found that the illness has been precipitated by such factors as an infection (commonly bronchopneumonia), pulmonary embolus, anaemia, cardiac arrhythmia, renal failure or even some overwhelming social crisis.

The diagnosis is sometimes difficult in the elderly if the cardinal sign of breathlessness is masked by confusion, agitation, nausea or coughing. There may simply be a history of the patient having become bedbound, incontinent and no longer able to cope at home.

Bilateral basal creps and ankle oedema are common in elderly persons who spend much of their time sitting in a chair, and the diagnosis of congestive cardiac failure cannot be made on these two signs alone. In addition there must be elevation of the jugular venous pressure: there may also be sacral oedema and an enlarged liver.

The signs in left ventricular failure may not be so clear-cut but there will usually be severe dyspnoea, particularly on effort, orthopnoea, paroxysmal nocturnal dyspnoea and evidence of left ventricular hypertrophy with a gallop rhythm.

Investigations

It is usual to take a chest X-ray to look for infection as well as enlargemnt of the heart or signs of pulmonary congestion (upper lobe blood diversion, peripheral oedema and Kerley B lines due to interstitial pulmonary oedema). The ECG should be examined for arrhythmias and signs of ischaemia. The haemoglobin, blood urea, creatinine and electrolytes must all be checked and also thyroid function measured if atrial fibrillation is present.

Treatment

Initially rest is advisable, but this may be in a chair rather than in bed. Where the patient is very ill and debilitated and the prospects for early

119

mobilization look remote, careful thought should be given to the use of anticoagulants to reduce the risk of deep vein thrombosis and pulmonary embolus.

Digoxin

The main indication for digoxin is to control fast atrial fibrillation. There is little point in giving it to patients with failure who are in sinus rhythm.

It is necessary to find out whether the patient is already taking digoxin since a loading dose given to someone who is digitalized is certain to produce toxicity. A convenient schedule is to give 1 mg digoxin on the first day and thereafter 0.25 mg a day: the aim being to control the heart rate. Because of (quite justified) fears of producing digoxin toxicity there has been a tendency to prescribe very small doses for all elderly patients. This is not always necessary and, indeed, means that some will be receiving a sub-therapeutic dose. Ideally, once stabilized all patients should have their plasma digoxin level checked to ensure that it lies between 1.3 and 2.6 nmol/l (1–2.0 ng/ml). Digoxin excretion is correlated very closely with renal function and a good estimate of the correct dose may be calculated from the creatinine clearance. Thus if glomerular filtration rate is 25 ml/min or more, serum urea less than 12 mmol/l (72 mg/100 ml) and serum creatinine less than 175 μ mol/l (2 mg/100 ml) it is safe to give a maintenance dose of 0.25 mg/day. If renal function is below this, a dose of 0.125 mg/day is reasonable. A dose of 0.0625 mg/day is unlikely to produce serum levels in the therapeutic range unless renal failure is severe (Roberts and Caird, 1976).

Digoxin toxicity

The patient may first complain of nausea and vomiting. Falls preceded by dizziness are sometimes the first indication of toxicity (Figure 1), and are the result of cardiac syncope due to arrhythmias. Toxicity should also be suspected in someone, previously in atrial fibrillation, whose pulse becomes slow and completely regular, suggesting complete heart block with a junctional escape rhythm (Hamer,

1976). Patients on digoxin whose pulse rate falls below 60 beats/min should miss a dose. Occasional ventricular ectopics may be tolerated but not when they regularly alternate (bigeminy). Atrial tachycardia with 2:1 or an irregular block is a common toxic effect and can give false impression of a failure to control atrial fibrillation with the dangerous consequence that the dose may be increased.

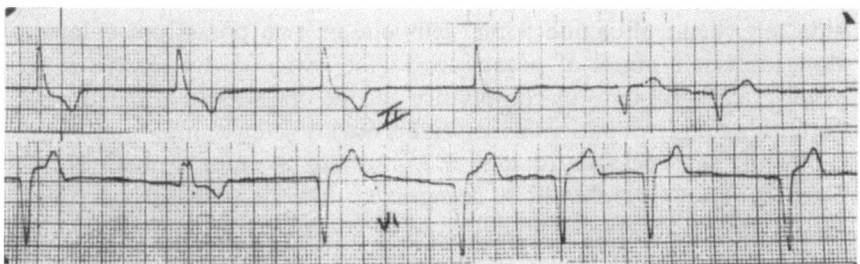

Figure 1 Electrocardiogram showing digoxin toxicity (serum digoxin 4·5 nmol/l) with bradycardia and frequent ectopics. The patient, a woman aged 84, presented with frequent falls preceded by dizziness. She improved considerably after the dose of digoxin was reduced.

When there are signs of toxicity, digoxin should be stopped and hypokalaemia corrected. Atrial arrhythmias do not usually need specific treatment but frequent ventricular ectopics should be controlled with lignocaine; an initial i.v. bolus of 100 mg followed by 1–2 mg/min through an i.v. drip. Beta-blockers are best avoided since they may potentiate the effect of digoxin and cause complete heart block.

Diuretics
These are the most valuable drugs. Within the broad categories of loop, thiazide and aldosterone antagonist diuretics there is a wide choice and only minor differences between drugs. It is best to familiarize oneself with one example of each and to limit one's prescribing to this small selection. Loop diuretics (frusemide, bumetanide) are potent, fast-acting and can be safely given in doses, for frusemide, of 20–80 mg once daily, for maintenance, or up to 1 g i.v. in renal failure. Some elderly patients find that they are too powerful and the

diuresis too swift, so that there is insufficient time to get to the lavatory. This rapid onset of action can be advantageous to poorly mobile patients who are given their diuretics when a relative or nurse is present to help them to the lavatory: thus their diuresis is over and done with for the day.

Thiazides are the most commonly used diuretic in maintenance therapy. Purists may advise that it is best to give a simple, cheap thiazide (e.g. bendrofluazide 5 mg) plus one or two potassium chloride slow tablets (8 mmol of potassium/tablet) twice daily. However, in practice the problems of compliance can be considerable. It is much better if a forgetful patient living on his own is given a single combined tablet of, say cyclopenthiazide 0.25 mg and 8 mmol slow-K (Navidrex K). Though it should be recognized that the potassium content may be insufficient.

Aldosterone antagonists (spironolactone, triamterene, amiloride) block or reverse the distal tubular sodium–potassium exchange. There is a small rise in plasma aldosterone in untreated congestive cardiac failure and this is the rationale for using aldosterone antagonists. An additional advantage of their use over potassium supplements is an increase in the labile cellular potassium pool. Spironolactone may be prescribed on its own or combined with a thiazide diuretic in a dose of 25 mg three times daily. A useful combination is hydrochlorothiazide 50 mg and amiloride 5 mg (Moduretic). Potassium supplements should not be given because of the risk of hyperkalaemia.

Potassium
It is said that a patient on diuretics needs potassium supplements of between 16 and 48 mmol/day to prevent hypokalaemia and its familiar consequences of tiredness, muscular weakness and enhancement of digoxin toxicity. There has, however, been some controversy about the need for supplements since total-body potassium counts appear to be unaltered by diuretics. Among geriatricians there is additional controversy over the relationship between age, potassium status and muscle strength.

It seems that in old age cardiac failure has a minor though significant effect upon potassium status (potassium deficit of 13.3% in patients treated with diuretics compared with controls), although there is no relationship between potassium dosage and total body potassium status (Ibrahim *et al.*, 1978). It was also found that potassium status, measured as the total-body potassium : free fat mass ratio, declines with age, even in healthy elderly people with normal diets. There are, as yet, no firm guidelines but it is probable that in relatively healthy old people potassium supplements are unnecessary. In ill patients, however, it is perhaps safer to continue with their use.

Patients who fail to respond
Patients with heart failure who do not respond to the usual treatment may have underlying disorders which should be looked for: chest infection, pulmonary embolus, hyponatraemia, thyrotoxicosis, digoxin toxicity or infective endocarditis.

When to stop treatment
The dangers of digoxin are well known, but even diuretics can cause troublesome side-effects such as incontinence, hyponatraemia, hypokalaemia and worsening of diabetes mellitus. Thus there are advantages in stopping both drugs when they are no longer needed. Very few patients need maintanance doses of either digoxin or diuretics and particularly with patients in hospital, no opportunity should be lost to stop these drugs to see if they are still needed (Burr *et al.*, 1977).

Pulmonary oedema
This is treated along the usual lines with morphine 5–10 mg, if the diagnosis of left ventricular failure is certain, or with aminophylline 250 mg given slowly i.v. if there is a possibility of obstructive airways disease. A small dose of frusemide (10 mg) i.v. will usually give a good diuresis and prompt relief. For elderly men with prostatic hypertrophy a catheter may be needed to prevent acute retention of urine. A salbutamol inhaler and high concentrations of oxygen may also be used, though the oxygen concentration should be reduced to 24 or 28% in the presence of obstructive airways disease.

COR PULMONALE

Right ventricular hypertrophy develops as a result of increased pulmonary blood flow, commonly due to chronic bronchitis, with or without emphysema.

Typically there is a history of chronic bronchitis with an acute episode of confusion, dyspnoea and wheezing, precipitated by a chest infection. The patient is centrally cyanosed with warm extremities, the jugular venous pressure is raised and the heart sounds are usually faint although a loud pulmonary second sound and a third heart sound may be heard. The ECG is often normal but may show right ventricular hypertrophy.

The acute episode is treated with controlled oxygen through a ventimask, physiotherapy, aminophylline 250 mg slowly i.v. and antibiotics.

VALVULAR HEART DISEASE

Rheumatic heart disease is still seen in the elderly although its frequency is declining. The incidence in elderly hospital patients was estimated by Bedford and Caird (1960) to be about 4%, which was a little higher than in the general population.

Aortic valve disease

This condition is common and stenosis is usually due to degeneration, fibrosis and calcification (wear and tear) in a tricuspid valve (Roberts, 1970). Aortic incompetence may be the result of rheumatic fever, calcification or syphilis, but dilatation of the aortic valve is frequently due to medial necrosis and elastin fragmentation of the aortic wall (Schlatmann and Becker, 1977).

124

Cardiovascular system

Mitral valve disease

This may be rheumatic in origin but most cases of mitral incompetence are due to ruptured chordae tendinae which is secondary either to ischaemia or to age-related degeneration. Elderly patients tolerate cardiac surgery well and the indications for surgery should be the same as for any other age group (de Bono, English and Milstein, 1978).

Heart murmurs

Systolic murmurs are found in up to 60% of elderly persons and are usually of the ejection type (*Br. Med. J.*, Leader, 1968). Very few of these murmurs can be regarded as being benign since there is a marked increase in the association of clinical cardiovascular abnormalities in patients with a systolic murmur compared with those without a murmur. The abnormalities found are cardiac failure, ischaemic heart disease, arrhythmias, hypertension, peripheral vascular disease and anaemia. Only 8% of patients with a systolic murmur have none of these conditions (Griffiths and Sheldon, 1975).

It is often difficult to decide whether an aortic ejection murmur is due to stenosis or sclerosis. In stenosis the murmur is usually loud, the second sound soft or absent and the left ventricle is hypertrophied. It is probable that aortic stenosis is under-diagnosed in the elderly and the aortic ejection systolic murmur dismissed as being unimportant. However, Pomerance (1968) found at necropsy that the aortic valve was normal in many of these patients and instead they had mitral incompetence due either to mitral ring calcification or to mucoid degeneration of the cusps.

INFECTIVE ENDOCARDITIS

Despite improvements in treatment the prognosis, particularly in the elderly, remains poor: the overall mortality is about 30%. In recent years there has been a rise in the age incidence so that now the majority of patients are over the age of 50 (Hayward, 1973). An increasing number of patients have underlying arteriosclerotic disease whilst the incidence of rheumatic heart disease has fallen.

Clinical features

Usually the onset is insidious with tiredness and general malaise. The presence of confusion and focal neurological signs due to small cerebral emboli may give the impression that the patient is suffering from multi-infarct dementia. The diagnosis is still based on the classical features of heart disease, fever, emboli and a positive blood culture. Because more elderly people are nowadays affected it is more common to find involvement of the aortic valve and pre-existing atrial fibrillation, formerly regarded as rare.

Clubbing, if present, is a valuable confirmatory finding, but Osler's nodes are rare and petechiae and splinter haemorrhages are not of diagnostic significance.

Investigations

The diagnosis must be considered in any patient with a heart murmur and pyrexia and blood taken for culture, three or four times over a period of 2–3 days. More cultures spread over a longer time are unlikely to be positive if the earlier ones are negative. Microscopic haematuria is almost invariable but there are no other specific laboratory tests. The ESR is usually raised and there may be mild anaemia with a normal or high leukocyte count.

Treatment

Although *Strep. viridans* is still the major organism responsible it is becoming increasingly common to find non-haemolytic streptococci, enterococci, and staphylococci. Penicillin is the drug of choice in *Strep. viridans* infections but in no other disease is it so vital to be guided by the bacteriologist both on the choice of antibiotic and the dosage.

Death is usually due to heart failure, either myocardial or valvular. Abrupt disintegration of the valve causes intense dyspnoea, low output state and low diastolic pressure. Urgent surgery should certainly be considered for these patients.

ARRHYTHMIAS AND CONDUCTION DEFECTS

In a random survey of the elderly Kennedy and Caird (1972) found occasional ectopics in about one-sixth of the subjects. Frequent ectopics (more than four in 40 complexes) were present in 4.5% and atrial fibrillation in 2.5%. The incidence of atrial fibrillation in sick elderly inpatients rises to 21.6% (Patel, 1977).

Abrupt changes of rhythm in an elderly person can lead to cardiac syncope, falls, transient ischaemic attacks and possibly even dementia. Arrhythmias should be suspected as the cause of a fall, particularly if it is preceded by dizziness and not related to a change in posture. In about half of these patients the ECG is normal in between falls and in only a quarter is there good evidence of an arrhythmia or conduction defect (Van Durme, 1975). The diagnosis can often only be made with the help of continuous ECG monitoring on a portable tape recorder.

Atrial fibrillation

Where established this may be found with almost any type of heart disease. Transient episodes of atrial fibrillation are sometimes seen following myocardial infarction. Digoxin is given to control the heart rate (see page 120). Where there is some urgency, for instance in left ventricular failure with pulmonary embolus, then a beta-adrenergic blocker should be given (e.g. practolol 5 mg i.v.).

Atrial flutter

Full digitalization is needed to induce the 4 : 1 block that will produce a satisfactory ventricular rate. Often it is better to combine a lower dose of digoxin with a beta-blocker (e.g. propranolol 20 mg b.d. or one slow-release oxprenolol 160 mg tablet daily).

Ventricular ectopics

Most often these follow myocardial infarction. One can either give an i.v. bolus of 100 mg of lignocaine followed by 1–2 mg/min through an i.v. drip or use disopyramide, an i.v. bolus of 2 mg/kg slowly plus 200 mg orally and then 200 mg orally 8-hourly for 24 hours followed by 100 mg 6-hourly.

Sick sinus syndrome

This occurs most frequently in the elderly and is characterized by chaotic atrial activity, changing P-wave contours, bradycardia and runs of atrial and nodal tachycardia. The patient may be asymptomatic or complain of lethargy, malaise, dizziness, palpitations and falls due to cardiac syncope. Drugs may induce supraventricular tachycardia in patients with bradycardia and vice-versa. Pacing is effective and is the treatment of choice (Radford and Julian, 1974).

Atrioventricular block

First-degree heart block (prolonged P–R interval) is found in 2% of healthy elderly people (Kennedy and Caird, 1972) and can usually be safely ignored. Second-degree block is of more significance. It indicates coronary artery disease and there is the risk that it may go on to complete heart block. When the block is irregular the patient may have falls due to cardiac syncope.

Complete heart block may present with classic Stokes–Adams attacks where the patient loses consciousness, falls to the ground with an absent or very slow pulse. His face is initially pale but becomes flushed as he recovers. Alternatively asymptomatic bradycardia may be found on routine examination, there may be a history of falls, evidence of a recent myocardial infarct or signs of heart failure.

Treatment is with slow-release isoprenaline, up to 30 mg 6-hourly. Larger doses can cause ventricular tachycardia and if control is not satisfactory then a pacemaker should be inserted.

ISCHAEMIC HEART DISEASE (IHD)

This is the commonest type of heart disease in the elderly, the incidence increasing with age. Below the age of 50 men are more likely to die from IHD than women, but after this age the difference in mortality declines until at age 80 the death rate for the sexes is equal. It has been suggested that this change is due to men losing a risk factor around the age of 50; possibly related to a reduction in plasma testosterone concentration(Heller and Jacobs, 1978).

The prevalence of IHD in a random elderly population was studied by Kitchin, Lowther and Milne (1973) who found that a history of angina was given by 10% of the sample. The ECG abnormalities present were strongly suggestive of IHD in 6% and a further 24% had possible ECG changes indicating IHD. At 5-year follow-up of the same sample 28% had died (28% were certified as dying from IHD). Mortality from IHD was strongly related to specific ECG abnormalities at the start of the period (ST depression, T inversion and atrial fibrillation) and to systolic blood pressure (Kitchin and Milne, 1977).

Angina pectoris

This is not often complained of in the elderly but it can be recognized in the same way as in younger age groups. The pain may not be very severe but its nature, site, the presence of dyspnoea, association with exercise and relief by rest are typical. Angina, in a small percentage of patients, is due not to IHD but to aortic valve disease or hypertension. Aggravating factors (thyrotoxicosis, anaemia, obesity, etc) should be looked for and corrected. The mainstays of treatment are:

129

(1) Glyceryl trinitrate tablets which should be chewed or sucked during an attack, or better still, as a prophylactic before exercise that is known to cause pain;

(2) Beta-adrenergic blocking drugs, such as propranolol, which is started at 10 mg twice daily and the dose doubled every 3 or 4 days until relief is obtained or the heart rate falls below 60 beats/min (Short, 1978).

Myocardial infarction

Clinical features

The commonest presentation is with dyspnoea. The onset is sudden and in about half the patients there is a background of long-standing heart failure. Atrial fibrillation is a frequent accompaniment (Pathy, 1967).

Next in order of frequency (19%) is the classical form with constricting chest pain or epigastric pain; a previous history of angina is more common in this group than in any other. Other presentations are confusion, sudden death, syncopal attacks with loss of consciousness but free of pain, hemiplegia, sensation of vertigo and faintness, peripheral gangrene or increased claudication, palpitations and progressive renal failure with uraemia. The overall incidence of pain-free infarction was 73% in Pathy's series; 60% when confused patients were excluded.

Treatment

The severity and mortality of myocardial infarction increases with age, and elderly as well as younger patients who are admitted to hospital do better in coronary care units (Williams *et al.*, 1976). However the elderly patient with an infarct probably does as well at home as in hospital, and whether or not a patient is admitted to hospital or to a coronary care unit depends as much on the individual's social circumstances as on the availability of beds. Synchronized d.c. shock and immediate defibrillation can be as successful in elderly as in younger patients, and the decision to place a patient 'on call' should depend not on his age but on his general health and previous quality of life.

Pain should be relieved with pethidine or morphine and frequent ventricular ectopics suppressed with lignocaine, 100 mg i.v. bolus followed by 1–2 mg/min i.v. or disopyramide (for dosage see under Ventricular ectopics, page 128. A restless, confused patient is best sedated with diazepam 5–10 mg i.m. Bradycardia responds to atropine 0.6 mg i.v. but second- or third-degree heart block may require pacing. Digoxin may be needed to control supraventricular arrhythmias. Routine anticoagulants are of no help but they should be used if a patient, because of frailty, obesity or hemiplegia, is at risk of developing a deep vein thrombosis or pulmonary embolus.

An optimistic attitude and early mobilization are important in maintaining the patient's morale and keeping his sights firmly set on regaining independence.

HYPERTENSION

Because of the lack of well-controlled clinical trials there is still much debate about whether or not hypertension in the elderly should be treated. There are fashions in these things and there is currently a move towards treating levels of blood pressure that a few years ago would have been ignored.

Hodkinson and Exton-Smith (1976) found no correlation between mortality and either the diagnosis of hypertension or systolic and diastolic blood pressure. However, both the Framingham study (Kannel, Gordon and Schwartz, 1971) and the Edinburgh study (Kitchin and Milne, 1977) showed that hypertension increased the risk of elderly people dying from ischaemic heart disease. The risk was greatest with raised systolic levels and there was a particularly gloomy prognosis when high blood pressure was associated with ECG evidence of left ventricular hypertrophy.

In the past there has been a tendency not to treat raised blood pressure levels until there is evidence of organ damage seen on the ECG, in renal function tests, retinal blood vessels, or by the occurrence of a stroke. However, as Dall (1978) has pointed out, it is often too late if one waits for a stroke before treating hypertension. He found that hypertension was a factor in 66% of stroke patients compared with 13% in those without stroke. In stroke patients whose hypertension was treated the recurrence rate was 16%, compared with 56% recurrence in an untreated group after 5 years.

One of the reasons why treatment of elderly hypertensives has been avoided is that the older drugs such as guanethidine produce too sudden a fall in blood pressure and cause postural hypotension and even cerebral infarction. It is now possible, however, to bring about a very gradual reduction in blood pressure by starting with a thiazide diuretic and adding a beta-blocker (e.g. propranolol 20 mg twice daily or one slow-release oxprenolol 160 mg tablet daily). If there is bronchospasm beta-blockers should be used with caution: a selective blocker such as metoprolol is probably safer. Beta-blocking drugs may cause hypoglycaemia in patients with diabetes. If methyl dopa is used it should be started at 125 mg twice daily and the dosage increased by 125 mg every few days.

The aim is to gently lower the pressure over several weeks to around 160/95. There are no firm rules, particularly for patients whose systolic pressure is between 160 and 180 mmHg and diastolic between 90 and 110 mmHg, and one has to be guided by the individual response to treatment.

VENOUS THROMBOEMBOLISM

Deep vein thrombosis

Clinically there is pain deep in the calf or thigh, which is made worse by dorsiflexion of the foot. A tender, palpable thrombosed vein is sometimes felt and a red streak seen overlying it. Swelling of the foot distal to the block is usual.

Investigations
Clinical signs are a poor indication of the presence of either deep vein thrombosis or pulmonary embolus. Simple, reliable, non-invasive methods for detecting deep vein thrombosis are widely available, such

as ^{125}I-fibrinogen, measurement of serum levels of fibrinogen degradation products and thermography.

Presentation

The risk of developing ^{125}I-fibrinogen detectable thrombi after surgery is nearly twice as high in patients over the age of 60 compared with those between 40 and 59 years. Coon (1977) has identified a number of factors which increase the risk of developing thromboembolism:

(1) Past history of venous thromboembolism or physical signs of venous insufficiency.
(2) Advanced age when accompanied by immobilization for 1 week or longer.
(3) Obesity.
(4) Recent hemiplegia or other cause of immobility.
(5) Heart disease: the risk is increased with severity of the heart disease and particularly in the presence of an arrhythmia or congestive cardiac failure.
(6) Carcinoma of the lung, gastrointestinal tract, genito-urinary tract and perhaps breast.
(7) Major operations, especially pinning of fractures of the neck of femur and abdominal surgery.

Early mobilization is the aim and the bedfast patient should frequently flex and dorsiflex his feet. However, where two or more of the risk factors listed above are present extra measures are needed. The possible courses of action include regular screening of the patient with ^{125}I-fibrinogen scanning; starting immediately with conventional heparin and oral anticoagulant therapy; or the use of low-dose calcium heparin. Calcium heparin 5000 units s.c. 2 hours before elective operation and then 8-hourly for 7 days reduces the risk of fatal pulmonary embolus (International Multicentre Trial, 1975). Dextran 40 is probably also effective in preventing post-operation thromboembolism (Gruber *et al.*, 1977).

Treatment
Heparin 10 000 units i.v. 6-hourly should be started immediately and the first dose of warfarin given. 15 mg of warfarin should be given on the first day, 10 mg on the second and thereafter the dose adjusted to keep the prothrombin time 2–2½ times normal; prothrombin times should be measured every 3 days. The elderly are especially sensitive to oral anticoagulants and maintenance doses may need to be as low as 1 mg of warfarin daily. Anticoagulants should be continued until the patient is fully recovered, usually 4–6 weeks.

In the acute stage the leg should be elevated and wrapped in an elastic bandage from toes to above the knee. Phenylbutazone 100 mg t.d.s. is effective in relieving pain, but if it is used the dose of warfarin will need to be reduced.

Pulmonary embolus

The prevalence of pulmonary embolus found at necropsy rises with age to 20% in those over 70 years. At all ages less than 10% of pulmonary emboli or deep vein thrombi are diagnosed during life.

Clinical features
There may be shock and circulatory collapse with massive pulmonary emboli or minor and rather non-specific signs when one of the smaller arteries is affected. Tachycardia is almost invariable; tachypnoea, raised jugular venous pressure, gallop rhythm, pleuritic pain and a pleural rub may be present. A sudden worsening of heart failure in a patient who appears to be recovering suggests a pulmonary embolism. Suspicion should also be high in poor-risk patients (*vide supra*) who deteriorate unexpectedly.

$S_1 Q_3 T_3$ changes are occasionally seen on the ECG, and chest X-ray may show a peripheral wedge-shaped shadow and blood diversion to the other lung.

Prevention and treatment of pulmonary embolus are as described for deep vein thrombosis.

PERIPHERAL VASCULAR DISEASE

Arterial insufficiency in the legs is usually the result of gradual occlusion by arteriosclerosis. It is often asymptomatic and only discovered at necropsy. Diabetes and cigarette smoking are known contributory factors.

Presentation is different in the elderly: rest pain or painless gangrene is commoner than intermittent claudication.

Rest pain

This is due to ischaemic neuritis but the distribution is not related to the dermatomes. It is often persistent, severe and worse at night. Some relief may be obtained by hanging the foot out of the bed. Peripheral pulses are absent and the toes may be red and tender with hyperaesthesia or paraesthesia. Occasionally, apart from absent pulses, the foot looks completely normal. Gangrene develops easily, particularly following trivial injury.

Treatment is directed towards improving the general health of the patient: correcting anaemia and dehydration, controlling heart failure, infection or diabetes and encouraging him to stop smoking. The leg should be cool whilst the rest of the body is kept warm, and the head of the bed should be elevated. Non-weight-bearing exercises for the leg are helpful. Relief of pain is vital and initially mefenamic acid (Ponstan) is useful; alcohol also helps. The pain, however, may be so severe that the patient's morale crumbles rapidly and opiates will be needed.

Surgical advice should be sought early since direct arterial surgery (endarterectomy or by-pass) may be very successful in an otherwise fit patient. Lumbar sympathectomy is often effective in relieving pain.

Ulceration

Ischaemic ulcers usually appear on the heels, toes or, where an arteritis is presented, as small lesions on the front of the leg. They are locally painful, pulses are absent and rest pain may be present.

135

Geriatrics

Lumbar sympathectomy may prevent the development of gangrene and reconstructive surgery may be indicated in selected patients. Hard, black sores on the heels are best left alone. They will take up to 12 months to heal, regardless of treatment.

Gangrene

This usually involves the toes, beginning as an area of purplish discoloration than then turns black. It often follows injury or interdigital fungal infections. If infection is avoided the gangrene remains dry and the toe may shrink and eventually drop off.

Amputation is all that the surgeon can offer although sympathectomy may allow a below-knee rather than a through-knee amputation. With a debilitated elderly patient it is often better to avoid surgery and control pain with adequate doses of opiates. However, with patients who are otherwise well, are not demented and do not have arthritis in the other leg, early operation should be advised in the expectation that successful mobilization will be possible.

Intermittent claudication

There is the familiar history of pain brought on by exercise and relieved by rest. Attention should be paid to the patient's general health and he should be advised to raise the heel of his shoe by half an inch to relax the gastrocnemius. Arteriography should be reserved for those who are likely to go on to surgery, and this is rarely indicated in patients over the age of 75 whose symptoms of arterial insufficiency are limited to intermittent claudication.

Embolus

Typically there is a sudden onset of pain in the limb, coldness, pallor and paraesthesia. Heparin 10 000 units i.v. should be given immediately and the surgeons contacted. Embolectomy will need to be done within 24 hours.

Amputation

A great deal of gloom, not all of it justified, surrounds this operation for both patient and surgeon. Statistics from 10 years ago showed that in an unselected group of patients a quarter would probably be dead within a year, a third within 2 years and two-thirds within 5 years. A patient surviving 5 years ago had an almost 50% chance of losing his other leg. Only a half of the above-knee amputees and three-quarters of the below-knee amputees would have been effectively rehabilitated (*Lancet* Leader, 1972). The general health of amputees is not good: over two-thirds have evidence of cerebrovascular disease (Little *et al.*, 1973).

Recently the proportion of below-knee amputations has risen considerably and this has had an important effect on the prospects for the amputee. At Roehampton, Robinson (1976) found that the hospital mortality for above-knee amputees was 36% and only 18% were discharged walking. The respective figures for below-knee amputees were 14% and 73%.

The patient should be carefully prepared before operation. Physiotherapy to strengthen the good leg, discussion with the occupational therapist and social worker and ideally, a visit from a patient who has already had an amputation and is successfully walking and independent.

The problems of tiring journeys to limb-fitting centres and long delays before the limb is available are well known. One way of avoiding the consequent loss of morale and mobility is to start walking exercises soon after operation using an early walking aid (Devas, 1977). Many patients find the usual artificial leg too heavy, and lighter limbs are now available. Some patients prefer to stick to their pylon. Where there is a skilled team and a mood of optimism the prospects for the elderly amputee regaining independence are good.

GIANT CELL ARTERITIS (TEMPORAL ARTERITIS)

The majority of patients are over the age of 70 and women outnumber men by about three to one. It is a multisystem disorder and characterized by a necrotic granulomatous reaction which mainly affects the media but also involves the intima and causes narrowing of the lumen.

Clinical features

The commonest presentations are headache, hyperalgesia of the scalp, pain on chewing and neck stiffness (Turner *et al.*, 1974). Visual symptoms (loss of vision or blurred vision), anorexia and weight loss are usual. Examination of the fundi shows either an ischaemic papillopathy or central retinal occlusion. Symptoms of polymyalgia rheumatica may also be present.

Investigations

The ESR is nearly always over 40 mm/h, and about a third of patients are anaemic. Nearly half will have a raised leukocyte count. Temporal artery biopsy will confirm the diagnosis.

Treatment

There should be no delay in starting oral prednisolone 40–60 mg/day. Symptoms often subside within 2 days and in 90% of patients the ESR will have returned to normal in 1 month. Turner *et al.* found that in patients who presented with visual disturbances this improved in 23%, remained unchanged in 64% and deteriorated in 13%. The longer the delay in starting steroids the greater the risk of blindness. Steroids are continued in lower doses for 6 months to a year, the aim being to keep the ESR low and the patient symptom-free. Long-term steroid therapy is hazardous in the elderly and azathiaprine may be used together with a low dose of prednisone or instead of it.

CARDIAC AMYLOID

In an unselected group of elderly subjects at necropsy cardiac amyloidosis was found in nearly 50%. In almost half of these cases amyloid

138

deposits were scanty and confined to the atrium. The prevalence and severity rises with age and is higher in women. There is a significant correlation between cardiac amyloidosis and the occurrence of atrial fibrillation and heart failure (Hodkinson and Pomerance, 1977).

ABDOMINAL ANEURYSM

The incidence of this condition continues to rise. It is largely confined to the elderly and can be very difficult to diagnose. A recent study (MacGregor, 1976) on unoperated ruptured abdominal aortic aneurysms found that the clinical history was usually short. Three-quarters had acute abdominal pain and just under a half had a pulsatile abdominal mass. It may be misdiagnosed as acute intestinal obstruction or pancreatitis but if suspected the patient should have a lateral abdominal X-ray or ultrasound.

Out of 41 cases the diagnosis was completely missed in 24. It was considered at necropsy that resection would have been technically possible without undue difficulties in the majority of cases. Therefore these patients should not be denied surgery.

REFERENCES

Bedford, P. D. and Caird, F. I. (1960). *Valvular Disease of the Heart in Old Age*. (London: J. & A. Churchill)

Br.Med.J., Leader, (1968). Systolic murmurs in the elderly. *Br.Med.J.*, **4**, 530

Burr, M. L., King, S., Davies, H. E. F. and Pathy, M. S. (1977). The effects of discontinuing long term diuretic therapy in the elderly. *Age and Ageing*, **6**, 38

Coon, W. W. (1977). Epidemiology of venous thromboembolism. *Ann. Surg.*, **186**, 149

Dall, J. L. C. (1978). *Mod.Med.Hypertension*, Suppl. 37

de Bono, A. H. B., English, T. A. H. and Milstein, B. B. (1978). Heart valve replacement in the elderly. *Br.Med.J.*, **2**, 917

Devas, M. (1977). The geriatric amputee. In M. Devas (ed.), *Geriatric Orthopaedics*. (London: Academic Press)

Gerstenblith, G., Lakatta, E. G. and Weisfeldt, M. L. (1976). Age changes in myocardial function and exercise response. *Prog.Cardiovasc.Dis.*, **19**, 1

Griffiths, R. A. and Sheldon, M. G. (1975). The clinical significance of systolic murmurs in the elderly. *Age and Ageing*, **4**, 99

Gruber, U. F., Duckert, F., Fridrich, R., Torhorst, J. and Rem, J. (1977). Prevention of postoperative thromboembolism by dextran 40, low dose heparin or xanthinol nicotinate. *Lancet*, **i**, 207

Hamer, J. (1976). Diseases of the cardiovascular system: cardiac failure. *Br.Med.J.*, **2**, 220

Hayward, G. W. (1973). Infective endocarditis: a changing disease. *Br.Med.J.*, **2**, 706 and 764

Heller, R. F. and Jacobs, H. S. (1978). Coronary heart disease in relation to age, sex and the menopause. *Br.Med.J.*, **1**, 472

Hodkinson, H. M. and Exton-Smith, A. N. (1976). Factors predicting mortality in the elderly in the community. *Age and Ageing*, **5**, 110

Hodkinson, H. M. and Pomerance, A. (1977). The clinical significance of senile cardiac amyloidosis: a prospective clinico-pathological study. *Q. J. Med.*, NS **46**, 381

International Multicentre Trial (1975) Prevention of fatal postoperative pulmonary embolism by low doses of heparin. *Lancet*, **ii**, 45

Ibrahim, I. K., Ritch, A. E. S., MacLennan, W. J. and May, T. (1978). Are potassium supplements for the elderly necessary? *Age and Ageing*, **7**, 165

Kannel, W. B., Gordon, T. and Schwartz, M. J. (1971). Systolic versus diastolic blood pressure and risk of coronary heart disease. *Am.J.Cardiol.*, **27**, 335

Kennedy, R. D. and Caird, F. I. (1972). The application of the Minnesota code to population studies of the electrocardiogram in the elderly. *Geront.Clin.*, **14**, 5

Kitchin, A. H., Lowther, C. P. and Milne, J. S. (1973). Prevalence of clinical and electrocardiographic evidence of ischaemic heart disease in the older population. *Br.Heart J.*, **35**, 946

Kitchin, A. H. and Milne, J. S. (1977). Longitudinal survey of ischaemic heart disease in randomly selected sample of older population. *Br. Heart J.*, **39**, 889

Lancet, Leader (1972). The elderly amputee. *Lancet*, **ii**, 747

Little, J. M., Petritsi-Jones, D., Zylstra, P., Williams, R. and Kerr, C.

(1973). A survey of amputations for degenerative vascular disease. *Med.J.Austral.*, **1**, 329

MacGregor, J. C. (1976). Unoperated ruptured abdominal aortic aneurysms: a retrospective clinico-pathological study over a 10 year period. *Br.J.Surg.*, **63**, 113

Patel, K. P. (1977). Electrocardiographic abnormalities in the sick elderly. *Age and Ageing*, **6**, 163

Pathy, M. S. (1967). Clinical presentation of myocardial infarction in the elderly. *Br.Heart J.*, **29**, 190

Pomerance, A. (1965). Pathology of the heart with and without cardiac failure in the aged. *Br.Heart J.*, **27**, 697

Pomerance, A. (1968). Cardiac pathology and systolic murmurs in the elderly. *Br.Heart J.*, **30**, 687

Radford, D. J. and Julian, D. G. (1974). Sick-sinus syndrome: experience of a cardiac pacemaker clinic. *Br.Med.J.*, **3**, 504

Roberts, W. C. (1970). The structure of the aortic valve in clinically isolated aortic stenosis. *Circ.*, **42**, 91

Roberts, M. A. and Caird, F. I. (1976). Steady-state kinetics of digoxin in the elderly. *Age and Ageing*, **5**, 214

Robinson, K. P. (1976). Long posterior flap amputation in geriatric patients with ischaemic disease. *Ann.R.C.Surg. Eng.*, **58**, 440

Schlatmann, T. J. M. and Becker, A. (1977). Histologic changes in the normal ageing aorta: implications for dissecting aortic aneurysm. *Am.J.Cardiol.*, **39**, 13

Short, D. (1978) Angina. *Br.Med.J.*, **2**, 939

Turner, R. G., Friedmann, A. I., Henry, J. and James, D. G. (1974). Giant cell arteritis. *Postgrad.Med.J.*, **50**, 265

Van Durme, J. P. (1975). Tachyarrhythmias and transient cerebral ischaemic attacks *Am.Heart J.*, **89**, 538

Williams, B. O., Begg, T. B., Semple, T. and McGuinness, J. B. (1976). The elderly in a coronary unit. *Br.Med.J.*, **2**, 451

7
Respiratory system

On gross examination the lungs of older people are lighter, whilst microscopically the thickness of the alveolar wall is reduced and the number of capillaries is decreased. Although there is no loss in the total number of alveoli they are increased in size with a reduction in the thickness of the elastic fibres in the bundles surrounding the alveolar ducts. The normal function of the elastic tissue is to maintain the patency of the small airways and this is impaired in old age.

It is difficult to assess the effects of age alone on respiratory function owing to the high prevalence of chronic disease and the effects of smoking and atmospheric pollution. One survey of respiratory function in Seventh-Day Adventists has shown that there is a progressive fall in forced vital capacity (FVC) and a slightly more rapid fall in the forced expiratory volume in 1 second (FEV_1). Thus a small reduction in the ratio of FVC/FEV_1 occurs during adult life, from a mean of 83% at the age of 20 to 68% at the age of 70. The residual volume (RV) increases with age, but the total lung capacity (TLC) shows little change, so that with advancing age RV occupies an increasing proportion of TLC. The alveolar–arterial oxygen gradient increases with age, probably owing to the fact that many alveoli remain closed and unventilated except during deep breathing.

143

Some of the effects of these physiological changes with age are that elderly people become breathless on exertion far more readily than younger individuals even in the absence of pulmonary disease, and the ability of the ventilatory system to respond to increased demands of respiratory infection is greatly diminished. Owing to the increase in kyphosis and in the rigidity of the chest wall the chests of old people tend to assume the position of inspiration with diminished movement. The percussion note is more tympanitic and extends over the area of cardiac and liver dullness. The breath sounds are weaker due to the diminished ventilatory air flow.

CHRONIC OBSTRUCTIVE AIRWAYS DISEASE

Chronic obstructive airways disease is the result of two pathological processes: chronic bronchitis and emphysema. These conditions are distinct entities which usually occur together; they probably result from common causes. Emphysema is defined as an increase in the size of air spaces distal to the terminal bronchiole with destructive changes in the walls. When emphysema predominates arterial oxygen tension is maintained by hyperventilation and the main complaint is breathlessness ('pink puffer'). Chronic bronchitis is arbitrarily defined on the basis of increased sputum production. The underlying processes are hypersecretion of mucus, which predisposes to pulmonary infections, and airways obstruction. The complaints are cough productive of sputum and recurrent chest infection. The underventilation, which is a feature of this condition, leads to cyanosis and polycythaemia ('blue bloater'). The majority of patients have both chronic bronchitis and emphysema and the clinical manifestations fall between the extreme ends of the spectrum.

The peak incidence of chronic bronchitis in the population occurs about the age of 50, but the prevalence of established conditions continues to rise in later life. It has been estimated that one million people in the United Kingdom are affected. It is more common in men than in women and about seven times more frequent in social class V than in social class I. These differences have been ascribed to such factors as

144

cigarette smoking, air pollution, occupation and living conditions.

Clinical features

Most elderly patients with chronic bronchitis and emphysema have reached a late stage of the disease and manifestations of airways obstruction are present:

Cough and expectoration

Chronic bronchitis is commonly spoken of as 'the winter cough of the aged'. It may occur only in the winter months, but later in life it is present throughout the year. It is made worse by sudden changes of temperature which occur when the patient moves from a warm room to the cold outside air; it is also aggravated by physical exertion and by change in position, especially when rising in the morning.

Dyspnoea

An increased respiratory rate with diminution in depth of respiration is almost constant even when the patient is at rest. At the time of onset of dyspnoea the FEV_1 is reduced within the range of 1.5–2.0 l, and there is a progressive fall of the FEV_1 to less than 1.0 l, by which time severe disability is present. The FEV_1 and its rate of fall is a good guide to prognosis.

Cyanosis

This is usually marked due to central anoxia and the development of secondary polycythaemia which is most marked in the 'blue bloater'. The haemoglobin value is rarely above 18 g/100 ml. The extremities are usually warm and the pulse strong.

Mental symptoms

Symptoms of cerebral depression are common in the elderly especially when anoxia is increased by an acute exacerbation of bronchitis, by bronchopneumonia or by the development of cardiac failure. The manifestations include giddiness, anorexia, nausea, insomnia, irritability, mental confusion and disorientation. The mental and behaviour disturbances may be so pronounced as to simulate dementia.

Respiratory failure

In a patient with long-standing cough and dyspnoea respiratory failure usually starts abruptly during a respiratory tract infection. Clinical indications of the onset are increasing lethargy, somnolence, headache, development of oedema, muscular twitching and myoclonic jerking of the limbs. Sometimes, confusion and stupor progressing to coma are more marked than breathlessness.

Diagnosis

The diagnosis is readily made in most cases; it is important to consider also the possibility of late-onset asthma as a cause of chronic airways disease. The main differentiation is from conditions causing the restrictive pulmonary syndrome. In the elderly these include: left ventricular failure, fibrosing alveolitis, rheumatoid disease of the lung, severe kyphoscoliosis and less often sarcoidosis and systemic lupus erythematosus. The distinction can usually be made clinically, and confirmed by the results of pulmonary function tests; the patient may be dyspnoeic but cyanosis is absent and there is no evidence of airways obstruction.

Management

The general measures include minimizing air pollution and discontinuing smoking. Patients with mild to moderate airways obstruction who give up smoking usually show a decrease in the rate at which lung function declines and some amelioration of symptoms. Simple measurements of peak expiratory flow rate, by means of a Wright flowmeter and of FEV_1, can be used to assess progress of the disease and response to treatment. Vaccination in the winter months is recommended since the death rate in these elderly patients during influenza epidemics is high.

146

Respiratory system

Treating infection

Exacerbation of bronchitis often follows upper respiratory viral infections and are due to bacterial infection most commonly with *H. influenzae*. Prompt treatment with a suitable antibiotic is essential without awaiting the results of sputum culture. The antibiotics of choice are doxycycline 200 mg initially and then 100 mg daily (can be given in the presence of renal insufficiency); tetracycline 250 mg four times daily; co-trimoxazole two tablets twice daily; ampicillin 250 mg four times a day, and amoxicillin 250 mg four times a day. In very ill elderly patients with severe bronchial infection, chloramphenicol, in spite of its hazards, is a reasonable first choice and the results are often surprisingly good. Elderly people who suffer from chronic bronchitis and who are at home should keep a spare supply of antibiotic; such prompt treatment of exacerbations is in general better than long-term chemoprophylaxis. The onset of drowsiness or mental confusion is an indication for immediate admission to hospital.

Oxygen therapy

Severe hypoxia is dangerous and it leads to confusional states, worsening cardiac failure and ultimately to severe depression in respiration. Unfortunately, these patients are dependent on hypoxia for their respiratory drive since they are insensitive to carbon dioxide. The administration of oxygen causes further under-breathing and aggravates carbon dioxide retention. When the PaO_2 is above 50 mmHg, oxygen therapy is rarely necessary even though cyanosis may be present, but when the PaO_2 is less than 35 mmHg oxygen is usually essential. For intermediate levels of PaO_2, between 35 and 50 mmHg, a careful assessment of the need for oxygen therapy must be made. It is most likely to be required when there is cardiac failure, co-existing ischaemic heart disease or severe dyspnoea. It should be administered by a Ventimask at a concentration of 24% oxygen. Higher concentrations (28%) should be used in patients with relatively low $PaCO_2$ but severe reduction in PaO_2. Usually the adverse effects of oxygen causing hypoventilation can be recognized clinically (and confirmed by blood gas analysis) within a few minutes of starting therapy; sometimes, however, the effects develop insidiously over hours or days.

147

Bronchodilation
Objective tests of pulmonary function show that bronchodilators produce only a small improvement, although subjectively most patients appear to derive benefit. The most widely used are the B2 selective, beta-adrenergic agonist drugs such as salbutamol and terbutaline. They are administered as pressurized aerosols one or two puffs four times a day. In patients with severe respiratory failure who do not tolerate aerosols, the drug can be given more effectively by a mask incorporating a nebulizer. Some patients can be helped by the oral administration of choline theophyllinate 200 mg three times a day or by Phyllocontin which causes less gastrointestinal side-effects. Aminophylline can be given by intravenous injection or infusion.

Improving ventilation
Patients with severe respiratory failure may benefit from respiratory stimulants; nikethamide 2 ml together with aminophylline 250 mg can be given by intravenous injection over 2 min and repeated every 2–4 h. Regular attention from the physiotherapist is necessary to see that the patient coughs adequately and produces sputum. Sedative drugs which depress respiration, for example barbiturates and linctus codeine, must not be given.

Intermittent positive pressure ventilation is sometimes required if the above measures fail; the aims are to secure adequate oxygenation, especially when the $PaCO_2$ is rising, and to remove secretions by tracheal and bronchial suction. It is most likely to be successful in patients suffering from a reversible disorder causing cerebral depression such as intercurrent infection or inappropriate sedation.

PNEUMONIA

Pneumonia is an acute inflammation of the lung due to invasion by micro-organisms. The classical division into lobar and bronchopneumonia is of little practical value. Lobar pneumonia behaving in a typical manner may occur in robust old persons and is often due to *Strep.*

pneumoniae, but it is uncommon compared with the much more frequent bronchopneumonia. This term is used to cover a variety of pneumonic conditions, and in the aged it is caused by, or associated with, a mixture of organisms which are normally found in the respiratory tract.

Pathogenesis

The high incidence of pneumonia and the variations in presentation are determined by general bodily changes and by local changes in the lungs which are common in old age. General changes predisposing to pneumonia include physiological impairment of immune function, malnutrition, hypothermia, malignancy and other wasting diseases, all of which lead to diminution in resistance to bacterial infection. The local changes most commonly result from structural damage to the respiratory system occurring in chronic bronchitis and the accumulation of bronchial secretions which provide a fertile nidus for the multiplication of invading organisms. Such mechanical factors are probably of as much importance as 'infection' in the development of pneumonia in the elderly. The organisms are often of low pathogenicity, and invade the lungs from the nasopharynx.

Hypostatic pneumonia
This occurs in elderly patients long confined to bed, or in those enfeebled by severe illness. The limited respiratory movements of the chest wall and diaphragm, together with depression of the cough reflex, enable secretions to collect in the bronchi of the dependent parts of the lungs.

Localized atelectatic pneumonias
These conditions occur in acute respiratory infections. The obstruction of a bronchus by mucus causes atelectasis of the part of the lung it supplies; this area then becomes infected by organisms present in the mucus. Bronchial carcinoma often presents as a localized atelectatic pneumonia which may progress to a lung abscess.

149

Inhalation pneumonias

These are due to aspiration into the bronchial tree of infected or irritant material. They are prone to occur in conditions associated with prolonged unconsciousness (e.g. after a cerebrovascular accident), in oesophageal obstruction with regurgitation, and in pseudobulbar palsy with difficulty in swallowing.

Clinical features

The mode of presentation of pneumonia in the aged is usually insidious and rarely does it have specific features which enable an early diagnosis to be made. The older person may be walking about during the stage when consolidation is becoming extensive and his only complaint may be of increasing fatigue and general weakness. Fever and leukocytosis are quite often absent. Cough may be unobtrusive, and sputum may be difficult to obtain for culture in the early stages. In other instances, especially with pre-existent bronchial disease, the sputum may be purulent. Slight dyspnoea and a rise in pulse rate may be the main indication of chest infection but these signs are often overlooked. In many elderly patients with pneumonia mental symptoms dominate the clinical picture (see Chapter 3); these include disturbance of sleep often with drowsiness in the daytime, and sleeplessness, restlessness and mental confusion at night.

The physical signs are variable. There may be cyanosis, rapid shallow respiration, and in the chest, impairment of percussion note, weak breath sounds or patches of bronchial breathing, and medium or fine rales over localized areas often with rhonchi audible over the whole of the chest. The areas where local signs are found may be small or may include the greater part of the lung bases. Sometimes all local signs of pneumonic consolidation are obscured by bronchitis and emphysema. Chest infections quite often precipitate congestive cardiac failure; on the other hand, left ventricular failure with congestion and oedema of the lung bases may predispose to the development of bronchopneumonia. In these cases it is difficult to distinguish between the two conditions.

Although the development of pneumonia in old age is usually

insidious, in some cases the onset is abrupt with early manifestations of respiratory failure such as cyanosis, drowsiness and mental confusion. Respiratory failure is more likely in patients with pre-existent lung disease but sometimes it occurs in previously symptomless people with an unusually virulent infection. In old people who have been exposed to cold, signs of hypothermia may dominate the clinical picture.

Clinical variations

In a small proportion of older people pneumonia is the result of infection with specific organisms.

Pneumococcal pneumonia
This may present a clinical picture of lobar consolidation similar to that seen in younger people. Mental confusion and delirium are often prominent, whereas the classical features of pleuritic pain, cough, rusty sputum and fever are less obvious.

Staphylococcal pneumonia
This condition can occur with thick creamy yellow sputum and the appearance of small multiple cavities within an area of consolidation on the chest radiograph.

Friedlander's pneumonia
This is almost always confined in its incidence to people over 50 years. It may be acute in onset with severe prostation, cherry-red sputum and the development of cavities in the area of lobar consolidation. The chronic form with multiple thin-walled cavities at the apex can mimic pulmonary tuberculosis, although the cavities are smaller and more numerous and the examination of the sputum for tubercle bacilli is negative.

Diagnosis

It is desirable that both sputum and blood cultures should be carried out. Postero-anterior and lateral radiographs of the chest should be taken, together with an electrocardiogram for evidence of ischaemic heart disease. If the facilities exist, it is advisable to measure PaO_2 and $PaCO_2$, especially when a patient develops pneumonia secondary to chronic obstructive airways disease.

Treatment

The aims of treatment of pneumonia in the elderly are to eradicate infection, to correct hypoxia, to relieve distressing symptoms and to prevent complications.

Infections

Antibiotics should be commenced at the earliest possible moment — after cultures have been taken but before the results are available. The initial choice must be a broad-spectrum antibiotic to combat a variety of organisms (see Table 1).

Many elderly patients when admitted to hospital will have been treated at home with benzylpenicillin and the tetracyclines; in these cases ampicillin (or amoxycillin) or co-trimoxazole should be the first choice. One of these drugs should also be used first in the patient already in hospital, especially when he has chronic bronchitis and emphysema. Emergency treatment is required in the severely ill patient with intravenous gentamicin combined with either flucloxacillin or cephaloridine. Chloramphenicol is justified in seriously ill patients despite the risk of agranulocytosis, especially when there is a known infection with *H. influenzae*.

No changes in the antibiotic regimen should be made for at least 48 hours unless there is rapid deterioration in the condition when intravenous therapy should be instituted. As soon as the identity of the organisms is known and the antibiotic sensitivity determined from the results of sputum culture the appropriate antibiotics can be substituted. If there is no improvement in 4–5 days further sputum culture should be made in case there has been a change in the infecting organisms.

152

TABLE 1
CHOICE OF ANTIBIOTICS

Antibiotic	Dose	Indications – Contraindications
(1) Ampicillin	1 g 6-hourly	First choice, except in patients who have previously received these antibiotics and have not responded or have penicillin allergy
(2) Amoxycillin	500 mg 8-hourly	
(3) Co-trimoxazole	2 tabs 8-hourly	First choice in patients who have not responded to (1) or (2) or who have penicillin allergy
(4) Gentamicin + flucloxacillin	80–120 mg i.v. 8-hourly 500 mg i.v. 6-hourly	Fulminating pneumonia with respiratory failure; penicillin resistant *Staph.* and gram-negative organisms
(5) Gentamicin + cephaloridine	1 g i.v. 8-hourly	As for (4) but if penicillin allergy is present; also against *Staph. aureus* and *Strep. pneumoneia*
(6) Benzylpenicillin	0.5–1.0 mega-units i.m. twice daily	Only in *Strep. pneumoniae* infection in previously fit individual who has not received antibiotics
(7) Chloramphenicol	500 mg 6-hourly	Severely ill patients with chronic bronchitis; *H. influenzae;* Friedlander's bacillus

153

Hypoxia
The adverse effects of anoxaemia on cerebral function in the elderly must be corrected as soon as possible. The hypoxia usually results from occlusion of the bronchi by inflammatory exudate, pulmonary consolidation and localized atelectasis. Provided there is no airways obstruction oxygen should be given at 6 l/min through a well-fitting mask. If, however, there is elevated $PaCO_2$ due to chronic airways disease, oxygen has to be given in lower concentration through a Venti-mask at a sufficient flow rate to relieve cerebral anoxia without increasing the degree of carbon dioxide narcosis (see page 147).

Accumulation of secretions
Mechanical factors leading to the retention of secretions are of great importance in most cases of pneumonia in the elderly. When the general condition of the patient permits therapeutic percussion of the chest, breathing exercises and suitable posturing of the patient may be of considerable help in draining the affected part of the bronchial tree.

Relief of symptoms
Most drugs which effectively relieve pain or abolish exhausting cough also cause depression of respiration. Simple analgesics such as dextro-propoxyphene or pentazocine can be used for pleuritic pain. For the control of insomnia and daytime restlessness long-acting and powerful hypnotics, sedatives and tranquillizers must be avoided. The short-acting chlormethiazole 500 mg (half-life about 4 hours) can when necessary be given in most cases with safety.

Complications
Aspiration of pleural effusion may be necessary for diagnosis and for the relief of dyspnoea. Patients with congestive cardiac failure, which may be either pre-existent or precipitated by broncho-pneumonia, should receive treatment using measures described in Chapter 6. Respiratory failure requires treatment on the lines already described (see page 148). Hypothermia sometimes complicates bronchopneumonia (see Chapter 5) and is best treated with intra-venous antibiotics since when injected intramuscularly they are

poorly absorbed owing to the disturbance of the peripheral circulation.

The lungs can be involved in several auto-immune diseases and the commonest clinical disorder is interstitial pulmonary fibrosis or 'fibrosing alveolitis' (Scadding, 1964). This can vary in severity from small areas of basal reticulation to the acute fulminating Hamman–Rich type of picture. In many cases of interstitial pulmonary fibrosis the cause is unknown, but of the cases examined by Turner-Warwick and Doniach (1965) 49% had rheumatoid factor present. Other less common causes are systemic lupus erythematosus, scleroderma, dermatomyositis and Sjögren's syndrome, all diseases in which autoimmunity is implicated. The main clinical features are dyspnoea, cyanosis at rest or after exercise, showers of fine or medium crepitations over the lungs and finger clubbing. The typical reticular pattern will be found on chest X-ray.

When the changes of fibrosing alveolitis are found on a routine chest X-ray the patient may remain asymptomatic for years, and in other cases with symptoms the disease may be only slowly progressive. The acute cases, which are uncommon in the elderly, may respond well to corticosteroids. For the majority of patients, however, the response to steroids is not impressive, and there is no evidence that steroids alter the course of the disease (Livingstone *et al.*, 1964).

BRONCHIAL CARCINOMA

Bronchial carcinoma is the commonest of all malignancies and the peak incidence is between 65 and 75 years. There are four main histological types: squamous carcinoma, anaplastic small-cell ('oatcell') carcinoma, adenocarcinoma and large-cell anaplastic carcinoma. Cigarette smoking is an important aetiological factor in squamous and oatcell carcinoma.

Clinical picture

The manifestations of the disease in the elderly do not differ from those seen in younger patients. It can mimic disorders in many bodily systems.

Respiratory symptoms

Cough, sputum production, haemoptysis and chest pain are common. Breathlessness results from distal bronchial occlusion and it is exacerbated by repeated attacks of pneumonia. Since most lesions are centrally situated the whole lobe or lung may be involved.

Direct extension

The primary growth may extend to adjacent tissues causing superior vena caval obstruction, hoarseness due to recurrent laryngeal paralysis, Horner's syndrome, brachial plexus involvement, dysphagia, pleural effusion and pericardial infiltration.

Metastatic spread

Metastases have occurred by the time the patient presents in 80% of small-cell carcinomas and in about 50% of the other types. They may involve the lymph nodes, bone, bone marrow, brain, meninges, liver and skin.

Non-metastatic manifestations

The neuromuscular manifestations include polyneuropathy, proximal myopathy, a myasthenia-like syndrome, spinocerebellar degeneration and dermatomyositis. In the musculoskeletal system hypertrophic pulmonary osteoarthropathy is not uncommon; more rarely this disease may start as a symmetrical polyarthropathy resembling rheumatoid arthritis (see Chapter 14).

Hormonal manifestations

The secretion of polypeptides with hormone-like properties produces a variety of syndromes including: a condition resembling Cushing's

156

disease; inappropriate ADH secretion causing hyponatraemia (see page 238); gynaecomastia due to hyperoestrogenism; hypercalcaemia due to a parathormone-like substance and a carcinoid syndrome, producing flushing, due to 5-hydroxytryptamine secreted by the tumour.

Diagnosis

In the majority of cases a diagnosis can be made on a postero-anterior and lateral chest radiograph and by examination of the sputum cytology. In doubtful cases it may be necessary to carry out mediastinal tomography and bronchoscopy. In the presence of a pleural effusion, pleural biopsy can be performed. The main difficulties in diagnosis arise when a patient presents with metastatic lesions or with non-metastatic neuromuscular and hormonal manifestations in the absence of evidence of primary growth on chest radiography.

Treatment

The only hope of cure is complete resection in patients with early bronchial carcinoma. The patients selected for surgery will usually be those with squamous cell carcinoma (and less ofter adenocarcinoma and large-cell anaplastic carcinoma) when the general condition is good with no apparent spread and no marked decline in pulmonary function. Lobectomy or pneumonectomy is nearly always required, but occasionally limited wedge resection is possible. More often palliation is all that can be offered. Radiography may provide great symptomatic relief for superior vena caval obstruction, for cough, haemoptysis and chest pain, and from pain arising from metastases in bone, but it has no influence on the duration of survival. Cytotoxic therapy, using such agents as cyclophosphamide, vincristine, methotrexate and comustine, may be effective in reducing the size of small-cell carcinomas but survival is only prolonged slightly if at all. The palliative measures for distressing symptoms, when they cannot be relieved by radiotherapy or cytotoxic drugs, are described in Chapter 17.

PULMONARY TUBERCULOSIS

During the last 20 years there has been a considerable fall in the incidence and mortality of tuberculosis. This decline in the disease in Britain has coincided with the use of effective anti-tuberculosis drugs. Reduction in frequency of tuberculosis has, however, been much less amongst the elderly population. The continuing occurrence of tuberculosis in old people is probably related to the poorer social conditions, the presence of other debilitating diseases and possibly to a decline in previous immunity.

Tuberculosis is often overlooked in the elderly for two reasons; first, the possibility of such a diagnosis is not considered, and second, there may be few symptoms and signs even when lung involvement is advanced. Thus undiagnosed lesions affecting older people, especially men, who remain without serious disability, are a source of danger since they may be responsible for the spread of infection in the community for years. The elderly sufferer from chronic fibroid phthisis is now the most important endemic focus of tuberculous infection in our society.

Clinical features

In the fibrocaseous variety of pulmonary tuberculosis there may be a history of ill health over a long period. Both large and small thick-walled cavities are present and there is often considerable pleural thickening. Progression of the disease is slow and intermittent with exacerbations of such symptoms as cough, dyspnoea and general debility. These symptoms, together with haemoptysis and the susceptibility to respiratory infections, are often due to emphysema and bronchiectatic dilation which complicate the tuberculous lesions. In the fibroid variety there is usually no long history of respiratory disorder, the general health often remains good, and night sweats and other symptoms of toxaemia are remarkably absent. By the age of 60, however, well-marked emphysema with associated chronic bronchitis has usually

158

developed and as a result cough and dyspnoea become more pronounced. Pleural effusion, especially when unilateral and persistent, should be suspected as being tuberculous provided malignancy can be excluded. Frequently there is a failure to make a diagnosis of miliary tuberculosis in the elderly (Proudfoot, 1969). Repeated chest radiographs may be needed before the characteristic miliary shadows are seen. The presentation is often with a pyrexia of unknown origin, but the erythrocyte sedimentation rate may be normal. A valuable diagnostic sign is a negative tuberculin test which later becomes positive.

Patients with pulmonary tuberculosis may die from acute tuberculous pneumonia or from haematogenous dissemination, but much more commonly the terminal event is bronchopneumonia or heart failure.

Diagnosis

The diagnosis of pulmonary tuberculosis in the older patient is often only suspected when a younger member of the family develops the miliary or meningitic form of the disease. Haemoptysis is another presenting feature which may lead to the diagnosis, but cough, dyspnoea, fatigue, debility and loss of weight are often neglected by the older patient. The localizing signs in the chest are often obscured by emphysema, especially in fibroid phthisis. Chronic tuberculous infiltration shows on the chest X-ray as dense opacities usually in one or both upper zones; caseation may lead to cavity formation. The apparently old, healed, fibrotic lesions should not be assumed to be inactive until further examinations have been carried out. The diagnosis can be confirmed by the finding of acid-fast bacilli in the sputum on direct microscopy. Specimens should also be cultured and the sensitivities of the organism to anti-tuberculous drugs determined.

If sputum cannot be obtained examination should be made of material from laryngeal swabs or early morning gastric lavage. Pleural biopsy is only likely to be of value when pleural effusion is present.

Treatment

The results of treatment of tuberculosis have been rigorously assessed on the basis of well-controlled clinical trials and modern chemotherapy alone is now sufficient treatment in almost all cases. Treatment should start with three of the drugs shown in Table 2 for a period of at least 8 weeks, or preferably until the drug sensitivities of the bacilli are known, followed by two drugs thereafter (Seaton, 1978).

The first three drugs shown in Table 2 are usually well tolerated in the elderly. The optimum regimen is a 9-month course of rifampicin and isoniazid supplemented by ethambutol for the first 8 weeks. The use of para-aminosalicylic acid (PAS) has now been superseded by ethambutol, and streptomycin should only be used in the elderly in cases of known drug resistance and then in a dose not exceeding 0.75 g daily. Certain drugs, such as PAS, pyrazinamide and ethionamide, can be held in reserve but they are generally less effective and more toxic.

TABLE 2
FIRST-LINE DRUGS FOR TUBERCULOSIS

Drug	Dose	Main toxic effects
Isoniazid	300 mg daily	Peripheral neuropathy – rare
Rifampicin	600 mg daily (before breakfast)	Gastrointestinal disturbances, abnormalities of liver function, hepatitis
Ethambutol	25 mg/kg daily for first 8 weeks; 15 mg/kg daily thereafter	Gastrointestinal disturbances, rashes, fever; optic neuritis (test visual acuity regularly)
Streptomycin	should not exceed 0.5–0.75 g daily by i.m. injection	Eighth nerve damage, nephropathy and hypersensitivity reactions (monitor blood concentrations in the elderly)

The objectives of this regimen are to ensure rapid killing of the organisms, to reduce infectivity and to prevent the development of resistant strains. The main obstacles to success are the failure of many elderly patients to comply with a complicated drug schedule over long periods (see Chapter 16). Ideally all elderly patients should be treated initially in hospital, especially when the more toxic drugs are used. Following discharge home very careful supervision (daily or twice-weekly visits by community nurses) is essential for the elderly patient whose drug compliance is poor.

REFERENCES

Livingstone, J. L., Lewis, J. G., Reid, L. and Jefferson, K. E. (1964). Diffuse interstitial pulmonary fibrosis. *Q. J. Med.* **33,** 71

Proudfoot, A. T., Akhtar, A. J., Douglas, A. C. and Horne, H. W. (1969). Miliary tuberculosis in adults. *Br. Med. J.*, **1,** 273

Scadding, J. G. (1964). Fibrosing alveolitis. *Br. Med. J.*, **2,** 686

Seaton, A. (1978). Today's treatment: tuberculosis. *Br. Med. J.*, **1,** 701

Turner-Warwick, M. and Doniach, D. (1965). Auto antibody studies in interstitial pulmonary fibrosis. *Br. Med. J.*, **1,** 886

8
Alimentary system

Many of the age-changes which occur in the alimentary system are asymptomatic. They may, however, directly predispose towards the development of clinical disorders; for example, constipation and diverticular disease become increasingly common with age. The functional and structural changes associated with ageing include: impairment of the sense of taste; disorder of oesophageal motility; atrophic changes in the gastric mucous membrane and the development of achlorhydria; functional impairment of small intestinal absorption; increase in gastrointestinal transit time leading to constipation and faecal impaction; the development of diverticula at various sites, in the oesophagus, duodenum, jejunum and especially in the colon.

Diagnostic difficulties

The high incidence of these changes leads to difficulties in evaluation of symptoms and signs and in the distinction of benign disorders from serious underlying diseases. Indigestion, for example, may have an origin which is either functional or organic; thus it may be due to disorders outside the gastrointestinal system, to impairment of gastric

163

secretion and gastritis, and more important it may be the presenting manifestation of malignant disease in the stomach or colon. Symptoms of large bowel obstruction due to carcinoma may long be attributed to an exacerbation of the patient's habitual constipation. The symptom of dysphagia in the older patient nearly always indicates an organic lesion.

Almost all diseases which affect younger patients occur in the elderly. In this chapter attention will be drawn to those diseases which are especially common in old age and which often have atypical features. Some of these diseases will be classified according to the disorders of function which they produce.

MOUTH AND TONGUE

Diseases within and outside the gastrointestinal system can cause white or brown furring of the tongue. A high proportion of elderly patients in hospital show this appearance. It has to be distinguished from oral moniliasis (*Candida* infection) which is characterized by white patches on the dorsal surface of the tongue, the oral mucosa inside the cheek and the gums. The diagnosis should be confirmed by microscopic examination of scrapings taken from the white patches.

Ill-fitting dentures can cause changes in the surface of the tongue, fissuring and ulceration. These oral changes can contribute to malnutrition since the sufferer tends to avoid more nutritious foods which require chewing (see Chapter 9). Many dentures worn by elderly people are 25 or more years old and they no longer fit properly on account of gingival resorption and changes in the shape of the mouth due to cerebrovascular disease. Patients with Parkinsonism sometimes claim that their dentures become loose after responding to treatment with L-dopa. In general, patients who have had even partial dentures for many years tolerate the fitting of new dentures better than those who have to wear dentures for the first time in old age. Fissuring at the angles of the mouth is more often due to ill-fitting dentures than it is to angular stomatitis associated with riboflavin deficiency. Another important cause of ulceration of the tongue and the buccal mucosa is the irritation caused by retention of tablets in the mouth; this condition is particularly associated with the administration of emepronium bromide used for the treatment of urinary incontinence. Infection of the salivary glands, especially parotitis, is common in seriously ill patients where oral hygiene is poor. Usually there is a very satisfactory response to treatment with penicillin.

A shiny red tongue associated with atrophy of the filiform papillae occurs in certain nutritional deficiencies. The causes include deficiency of iron, vitamins of the B group (see Chapter 9), folic acid and vitamin B_{12}. In pernicious anaemia, although the classical red beef tongue is occasionally seen it is more often pale and smooth. Varicosity of the large vessels on the under-surface of the tongue gives rise to the common condition of 'mulberry' or 'caviar' tongue. They are due to changes in the supportive connective tissues and are probably of little clinical significance. Sublingual haemorrhages can occur in vitamin C deficiency but they have to be distinguished from the much more common lesions which Andrews and his colleagues (1969) have shown to be due to microvaricosities or aneurysmal dilatation of the small vessels on the under-surface of the tongue. They are not due to acute vitamin C deficiency but it is possible that they may be the result of a long-continued mild deficiency affecting collagen in the tissues.

DYSPHAGIA

The term dysphagia is applied when there is difficulty in initiating swallowing or when there is a sensation of food sticking anywhere between the pharynx and the stomach. The causes can be classified according to the level of the lesion. The patient's history is often of help in location of the level, although occasionally in cases of middle or lower oesophageal obstruction the symptoms are referred to a higher level. There are three main sites of obstruction in the oesophagus: the upper end, the level of the bifurcation of the trachea and the cardiac region; intermediate sites are less common.

Causes

1. Pharyngo-oesophageal obstruction

One of the commonest causes at this site is the neuromuscular incoordination which occurs in pseudobulbar palsy (see Chapter 4). Unlike other causes of dysphagia it is characterized by a greater difficulty in swallowing liquids rather than foods of a semi-solid consistency.

Two sites of carcinoma can lead to this type of dysphagia; they are carcinoma of the larynx, mainly in men, and post-cricoid carcinoma which is much more common in elderly women. In the latter there may be a history of the Plummer–Vinson syndrome due to lesions in the tongue and upper part of the alimentary system associated with iron-deficiency anaemia. The syndrome itself can cause dysphagia but it is more common in middle age and it is not often seen in women over the age of 65.

Diverticula occur at various sites and although rare are more common in the old than in the young. A diverticulum of the posterior wall of the pharyngo-oesophageal junction leads to difficulty in swallowing associated with gurgling in the neck; sometimes the swelling is palpable and it can be reduced by external pressure.

2. Mid-oesophageal dysphagia

Obstruction in the middle third of the oesophagus is usually due to carcinoma which at this site is 10 times more common in men than in women. Causes of external compression of the oesophagus are aortic aneurysm and unfolding of the aorta (dysphagia lusoria) and enlargement of the mediastinal glands when they are involved by neoplasm from such primary sites as the bronchus, breast, stomach and pancreas. Two rare causes of dysphagia associated with disorder of oesophageal motility should be considered. These are diffuse oesophageal spasm in which barium swallow may reveal 'corkscrew' oesophagus, or alternatively a complete absence of peristalsis, and rigidity of the oesophagus due to its involvement in scleroderma.

3. Lower-oesophageal dysphagia

The two major causes in this region are oesophageal hiatus hernia

166

(considered below) and malignancy. Carcinoma may arise in the lower end of the oesophagus or in the cardiac portion of the stomach. The onset is usually gradual with increasing discomfort on swallowing, but occasionally it is acute when a poorly chewed bolus of food becomes impacted. As in other causes of dysphagia the presentation can be pneumonia due to aspiration of food particles from the obstructed oesophagus.

Management

The diagnosis must be confirmed by means of a barium swallow examination. In the majority of cases this will localize the site of obstruction and will often help in the diagnosis of the cause. In 22% of the cases of dysphagia reported by Exton-Smith and Osborne (1961) radiology failed to reveal a cause. In these cases oesophagoscopy is essential; it is also often necessary in the differentiation of benign stricture from carcinoma. The primary cause should be treated wherever possible. If it is not amenable to treatment a lumen in the oesophagus should be maintained by means of a Mousseau–Barbin tube inserted at oesophagoscopy. The decision to pass a nasogastric tube must depend on the likely prognosis. In patients with a poor prognosis it may be of great help in relieving distress caused by choking and dehydration. Gastrostomy is rarely performed as it produces so much distress in itself.

OESOPHAGEAL HIATUS HERNIA

Hiatus hernia deserves special consideration because it becomes increasingly common with advancing age. When the presenting feature is dysphagia it has to be differentiated from carcinoma. There are, however, other diagnostic difficulties; the symptoms it can produce simulate those due to disease in other systems (e.g. ischaemic heart disease) and since it is so common the finding of a hiatus hernia should not lead the physician to attribute the patient's symptoms to it until other possibilities have been excluded.

167

Types of hiatus hernia

There are two main types of herniation of the stomach through the oesophageal hiatus of the diaphragm:

(1) The oesophagogastric (sliding) type: this is the more common form. The portion of the cardia which passes into the thorax is seldom of great size but the symptoms are often striking due to reflux oesophagitis.

(2) The para-oesophageal (rolling) type: the fundus of the stomach passes upwards in front of the cardia which remains at its normal level in relation to the diaphragmatic opening. As there is no sphincter disturbance reflux oesophagitis does not occur.

In addition there is a mixed type with features of the sliding and rolling types of hernia.

Clinical features

Symptoms are most striking when reflux oesophagitis is present.

(a) Symptoms due to oesophagitis
Dysphagia or pain felt at the lower end of the sternum whenever food is taken is often the most prominent symptom. It may be provoked by bending, stooping or lying down. In the majority of cases there is only mild pain but sometimes it is severe with widespread radiation to the back, the neck and down the arms. Dysphagia may also be due to oesophageal stricture consequent upon fibrosis associated with peptic ulceration of the oesophagus.

(b) Symptoms due to hernia
In para-oesophageal hernia the patient may experience retrosternal discomfort coming on at the beginning of the meal; relief may be obtained by walking about, and the patient can often continue the meal without further discomfort. Pressure from the hernial sac may irritate the diaphragm with the production of cough or hiccup. But even very large rolling type hernias can be asymptomatic.

(c) Symptoms due to haemorrhage

Bleeding may occur from peptic ulceration of the oesophagus or from associated gastric ulcer. Thus there may be frank haematemesis or melaena, and a progressive iron deficiency anaemia especially when there is a slow 'oozing' of blood.

Diagnosis

Barium meal examination will usually reveal the hiatus hernia and its type. When the appearances are those of stricture at the lower end of the oesophagus it is necessary to differentiate fibrosis due to oesophagitis from carcinoma in the region of the cardia. Oesophagoscopy is often necessary in these cases. The differentiation of substernal pain due to hiatus hernia from that due to ischaemic heart disease is sometimes difficult and the two may coexist. When the presentation is with anaemia it should not be assumed that the hiatus hernia is the site of blood loss until other causes of gastrointestinal haemorrhage have been excluded.

Management

Symptomatic relief is obtained in most patients by medical treatment. The patient should sleep with the head of the bed raised, avoid stooping and reduce the size of meals, especially those taken in the late evening. Weight reduction is desirable in the obese patient. Symptoms due to reflux oesophagitis can usually be controlled by adopting a similar regimen to that used in the treatment of gastric or duodenal ulcer. The histamine H2 receptor antagonist, cimetidine, should be given in a dose of 400 mg four times a day (with meals and at bedtime) for a period of 4–8 weeks. Gaviscon, a mixture of alginic acid, magnesium trisilicate, aluminium hydroxide gel and sodium bicarbonate, given four times daily after meals is useful in providing relief of symptoms due to reflux oesophagitis.

PEPTIC ULCER

Peptic ulcer can occur at several sites all of which are bathed in peptic juice. They include the lower end of the oesophagus, the stomach, the first and second part of the duodenum and the jejunum after gastroenterostomy. The incidence of gastric ulcer increases with age and in those over 75 it approximates to the incidence of duodenal ulceration. The clinical features of peptic ulcer may be similar in the elderly to those in the young; but in many cases, especially in gastric ulcer, the presentation may be atypical.

Giant gastric ulcer

The most striking difference in peptic ulceration between the old and the young is the frequent occurrence of benign giant gastric ulcer in patients over the age of 60. Strange (1963) has pointed out that ulcers over 5 cm in diameter on the lesser curve of the stomach are more often benign than malignant. They may be asymptomatic but in other cases the symptoms are vague pain in the epigastrium or left side of the chest, anaemia and weight loss. Sometimes the presenting manifestations are perforation, haematemesis or a fainting attack due to the loss of blood which is later passed as a 'tarry stool'. Although not malignant these ulcers are an important cause of death since massive haemorrhage may occur from erosion of an arteriosclerotic vessel in the base of the ulcer.

Complications of peptic ulcer

There are three main complications of peptic ulcer:

Haemorrhage

This may be acute, leading to haematemesis or melaena, or chronic, with a slow oozing of blood producing iron deficiency anaemia.

Alimentary system

Perforation

This may also be acute with the typical sudden development of severe epigastric pain and shock; often, however, it is sub-acute and the pain develops slowly, or the initial severe pain rapidly disappears after a few hours. In these cases the omentum or some viscus is adherent to the site at which perforation occurs.

Obstruction

This occurs mainly in prepyloric and duodenal ulcers. It is characterized by recurrent vomiting and loss of weight. Hour-glass contraction of the stomach is rare but it is occasionally seen in the elderly person who has had for many years an ulcer in the middle of the lesser curve.

Management

A barium meal is usually essential for diagnosis. The possibility of malignancy often cannot be excluded by this investigation alone and fibroscopy is necessary. In treatment bed-rest and a strict dietary regimen are not indicated. Soluble alkali should be avoided since uraemia may result from alkalosis when renal function is already impaired. Aluminium hydroxide gel is usually satisfactory; magnesium trisilicate can be added when there is a tendency to constipation. Carbenoxolone sodium can be of value in promoting healing but in the elderly regular surveillance is necessary since this drug can cause hypokalaemia, fluid retention and a rise in blood pressure.

The histamine H2 receptor antagonist, cimetidine, is now the treatment of choice and it usually leads to rapid healing of the ulcer. It should be given in a dose of 1 g/day – 200 mg three times a day with meals and 400 mg at bedtime. If there is inadequate symptomatic relief or evidence of continuing ulceration the dose can be increased to 400 mg four times a day. Treatment should be continued for at least 6 weeks and in many cases maintenance therapy is necessary with a reduced dose of 400 mg morning and evening. There is a danger of relapse when treatment is stopped and in some cases the drug must be continued indefinitely.

171

Complications of partial gastrectomy

Between 5 and 15% of patients who undergo partial gastrectomy for peptic ulcer develop complications. These may develop early after operation; for example, the dumping syndrome consisting of postprandial sweating, unpleasant warmth, flushing, nausea and abdominal fulness. This is probably due to the rapid passage of food into the proximal small bowel and the high osmotic pressure causes fluid to accumulate in the gut lumen. More serious are the late complications which occur particularly after a Polya gastrectomy. These are due to bacterial colonization of a blind loop with production of steatorrhoea. The manifestations are the result of nutritional deficiencies – osteomalacia due to vitamin D deficiency and iron deficiency anaemia due to impaired iron absorption. Megaloblastic anaemia may also occur owing to vitamin B_{12} deficiency when the intrinsic factor-producing area of the stomach is removed. Loss of weight occurs in almost all patients after partial gastrectomy.

MALABSORPTION SYNDROME

Intestinal malabsorption becomes increasingly prevalent in old age. Histological examination shows that the villi of the small intestine change their shape and become shorter and broader. This leads to a diminution in the area of absorbing surface. Some of these changes are 'physiological' and are to be regarded as part of the process of ageing. The extent to which small bowel ischaemia, due to mesenteric arterial disease, contributes to the villous atrophy with consequent impairment of intestinal function is at present unknown.

Causes

Price and his colleagues (1977), in a study of steatorrhoea in the elderly, found benign pancreatic disease to be the commonest cause in this age group. Other important causes include partial gastrectomy,

172

small bowel diverticulosis and other contaminated bowel syndromes, gluten enteropathy, amyloidosis, and certain skin diseases. In some very old people in spite of exhaustive investigations no cause can be found; it is possible that some of these cases are due to abnormal bacterial colonization which occurs more frequently in extreme old age and leads to a reduction of absorptive capacity of the mucosal cells of the jejunum.

Clinical features

Malabsorption syndromes may present with an increase in bowel habits. In steatorrhoea the increased fat content of the stools causes them to be bulky, pale and foul-smelling. Often, however, the clinical manifestations are outside the gastrointestinal system and they are due to nutrient deficiencies resulting from malabsorption. Anaemia is the commonest presenting disorder. It is usually microcytic, hypochromic due to iron deficiency, but it can also be macrocytic associated with deficiencies of folic acid or vitamin B_{12}. The malabsorption syndrome is an important cause of osteomalacia in old age (see Chapter 14) and is due to deficiency of vitamin D. Dent and his colleagues (1961) have drawn attention to the association between steatorrhoea and hypothermia.

Investigations

Many tests have been devised for the investigation of malabsorption. Those most often employed are:

1. Fat absorption
The fat content of the stools is measured and in steatorrhoea the faecal fat exceeds 17.5 mmol/day over a minimum of 5 days. The accuracy of the test depends upon the completeness of the faecal collection over this period of time and this is difficult to achieve in some elderly patients.

2. *Xylose absorption*

Measurement of the blood xylose level 1 hour after standard oral dose (5 g) is perhaps the most reliable single test of non-pancreatic malabsorption in the elderly. It is unaffected by mild impairment of renal function and is not correlated with age (Kendall, 1970). Urinary xylose, however, shows a steep decline with age because of physiological impairment of renal function.

3. *Iron absorption*

The serum iron levels are often low and following the oral administration of 100 mg ferrous sulphate the peak level of serum iron is less than 14μ mol/l. In many cases the iron-binding capacity (TIBC) is reduced and in others there is no expected increase to correspond with the iron deficiency. In general the decreased TIBC correlates with a reduction in serum albumin.

4. *Folate and vitamin B_{12} absorption*

Low levels of serum and red cell folate and of serum vitamin B_{12} are found in patients with malabsorption syndrome. Tests based on the absorption of these nutrients are unsatisfactory in the elderly. Impaired renal function and difficulties in urine collection limit the usefulness of the Schilling test in old age.

5. *Small-bowel biopsy*

A specimen of small intestinal mucosa can be obtained by means of a Crosby capsule. The main indication for this procedure is to confirm or exclude the diagnosis of gluten enteropathy.

6. *Bacterial flora*

Direct studies of bacterial flora in the small intestine are useful in conditions where stasis occurs, but they are difficult to carry out in the elderly. There is, however, a simpler indirect test; colonization of the small bowel with metabolically active bacteria leads to increased deconjugation of bile salts. These changes can be detected by measurement of the radioactivity of expired air following the administration of radioactively labelled [C14]glycocholic acid.

174

Alimentary system

Unfortunately there is no single screening procedure in malabsorption syndromes since the tests described will be of no value in the diagnosis of chronic pancreatitis.

Management

Only occasionally can the underlying cause of malabsorption be corrected and the patient will usually be treated by replacement therapy for nutritional deficiencies of iron, folic acid, vitamin B_{12} and vitamin D. Elderly patients with gluten enteropathy can sometimes be successfully treated by a gluten-free diet. In patients with blind loop syndrome and diverticulosis the bacterial overgrowth can be reduced by the administration of an antibiotic such as neomycin.

JAUNDICE IN THE ELDERLY

In a series of 80 patients, whose ages ranged from 65 to 89 years, it was found that the jaundice was obstructive in nature in 80% of cases, hepatic in 16% and haemolytic in 4% (Huete-Armijo and Exton-Smith, 1962). The findings of this study are summarized in Figure 1.

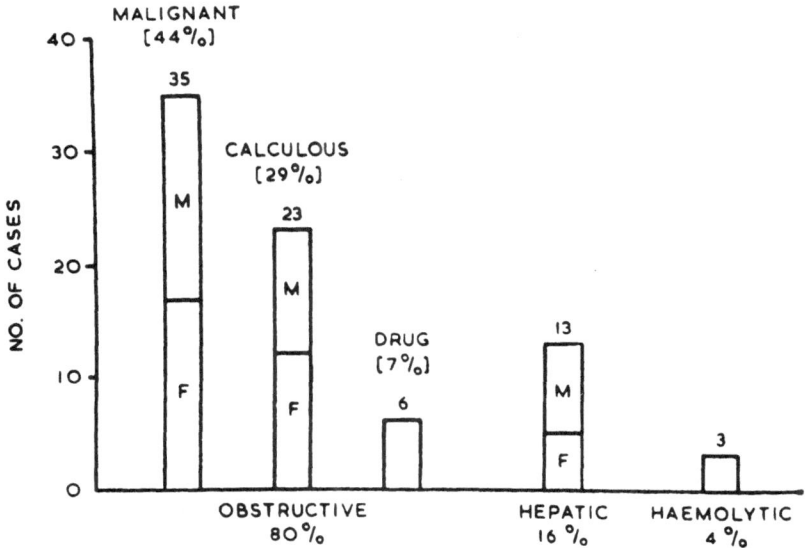

Figure 1   Types of jaundice

175

The commonest cause of neoplastic obstructive jaundice was carcinoma of the head of the pancreas followed by secondary carcinoma in the liver in which the primary was in the gastrointestinal tract in two-thirds of cases. Hepatic jaundice was most often due to viral hepatitis, followed by cirrhosis of the liver. Haemolytic jaundice, although uncommon in the elderly, can be due to blood disorders and drugs; in patients with congestive cardiac failure jaundice can develop as a result of pulmonary infarction because the anoxic liver cells are unable to deal with the increased pigment load liberated from haemoglobin.

The causes of the two most important types of jaundice – obstructive and hepatocellular – will be discussed in greater detail.

Obstructive jaundice

There are two types of obstruction: extrahepatic due to neoplasm or gall-stones and intrahepatic due usually to drugs causing cholestasis.

Neoplastic jaundice

Carcinoma of the head of the pancreas is the commonest cause of neoplastic jaundice. Although the classical description is of progressive painless jaundice, it is now recognized that pain occurs during the course of the illness in nearly half the cases. It is inconstant in nature and in its localization; it may be felt in the epigastrium, the right or left hypochondrium and frequently radiates to the back. It is variously described as being dull, aching, boring or burning in nature and is unrelieved by food or alkalis. The stools become clay-coloured and the urine dark, and these changes are persistent throughout the clinical course. In carcinoma of the ampulla of Vater, however, the intensity of the jaundice may fluctuate and the stools may have a metallic shiny appearance ('silver stool' sign), due to the presence of altered blood in the pale faeces.

The presence of a smooth, distended, non-tender gall-bladder is a valuable diagnostic sign of obstructive neoplastic jaundice. When, however, the enlargement of the gall-bladder is not detected on clinical examination carcinoma of the head of the pancreas or of the ampulla cannot be excluded.

176

The next most important cause of neoplastic jaundice is metastatic carcinoma in the liver or the lymph nodes in the porta hepatis. In two-thirds of cases the primary is in the alimentary tract or its appendages, but it may also be in other sites such as the bronchus, breast and urogenital organs. In many cases of metastatic carcinoma of the liver jaundice is absent; it is only severe in degree when there is obstruction of the main hepatic ducts at the hilum. The liver shows a hard nodular enlargement on palpation. In carcinoma of the gall-bladder there is often an antecedent history of gall-stones and the jaundice results from obstruction of the common duct either by compression or by direct extension of the growth.

Calculous jaundice

Although gall-stones are found at autopsy in about one-third of persons over 70 years of age biliary colic or jaundice only appear in a small proportion. Apart from a mild jaundice of short duration which may occur in acute calculous cholecystitis, the main cause of jaundice is impaction of a stone in the common bile duct. Obstruction is usually incomplete, or at least temporarily complete immediately after impaction; later the stone becomes loose in the duct, allowing bile to pass. The resulting jaundice is usually moderately intense and intermittent. Clinically impaction of the stone in the common duct gives rise to biliary colic in which the pain is situated in the epigastrium, either hypochondrium, the precordial region or between the shoulder blades. Rigors, fever and vomiting are frequent associated symptoms. Severe jaundice due to gall-stone impaction may occur in the absence of pain, and biliary colic occurred in only 7 of the 23 cases of calculous jaundice reported by Huete-Armijo and Exton-Smith (1962). It is in these cases that a diagnosis of neoplastic obstruction is often made.

Intrahepatic cholestasis

Most cases of intrahepatic cholestatic obstruction are due to drugs. The cholestasis is a hypersensitivity reaction and the drugs incriminated include: the phenothiazines (especially chlorpromazine), antidepressants, the benzodiazepines, oral hypoglycaemic agents, thiazide diuretics, phenylbutazone, antithyroid drugs and the sulphonamides.

After stopping the drug, recovery is usual in a matter of weeks. Rarely, the jaundice persists with the development of steatorrhoea, weight loss and osteomalacia. Such cases resemble primary biliary cirrhosis with high serum cholesterol and alkaline phosphatase levels, but the specific immunofluorescent test for biliary cirrhosis is negative.

Apart from drugs, atypical virus hepatitis must also be considered as a cause of intrahepatic cholestasis. Among the 28 patients with jaundice due to virus hepatitis, all of whom had an aspiration biopsy of the liver, Shorter and his colleagues (1959) found five cases of intrahepatic cholestasis.

Primary biliary cirrhosis
Although this condition occurs typically in middle-aged females it is also found in people over the age of 65. Pruritis and skin pigmentation are often striking; jaundice appears but sometimes only after many months or years. A malabsorption syndrome develops and osteomalacia is a common complication. Clubbing of the fingers also occurs. The liver is very large, firm and smooth and the spleen is often enlarged. Signs of portal hypertension and liver failure may develop. It is due to a chronic non-suppurative cholangitis. The presence of a positive mitochondrial immunofluorescent test and raised serum IgM levels help to differentiate the condition from extrahepatic biliary obstruction and from other intrahepatic forms of cholestasis.

Hepatocellular jaundice

The two main causes of hepatocellular jaundice are virus hepatitis and cirrhosis.

Virus hepatitis
Both forms of virus hepatitis, hepatitis-A and hepatitis-B, can occur in old age. Jaundice appears after a prodromal phase often prescribed as 'gastric flu' consisting of anorexia, nausea, abdominal discomfort and mild pyrexia. In the elderly the course is likely to be prolonged, with jaundice persisting for 6 weeks or more. Weight loss and mental

changes are common. Hepatitis-B has an even more insidious onset and prolonged course in the elderly. There is a relationship between hepatitis-B and the development of chronic hepatitis, cirrhosis and hepatoma (Dudley *et al.*, 1972).

Cirrhosis of the liver

The elderly patient may show the classical picture of a small fibrosed liver, ascites, portal hypertension and hepatic failure. The examination should include a search for 'spider naevi' and assessment of mental function for evidence of hepatic encephalopathy. Jaundice occurs in only about half the cases and is usually mild.

Diagnosis

The main difficulties in the differential diagnosis of the causes of jaundice in the elderly lie in the distinction between the following conditions.

(1) Carcinoma of the head of the pancreas from calculous obstruction especially when the impaction of the gall-stones in the common duct is unaccompanied by pain.
(2) The intermittent obstruction occurring in gall-stones and that due to carcinoma of the ampulla.
(3) Extrahepatic obstruction from intrahepatic cholestasis due to drugs.
(4) Virus hepatitis in which the cholestatic phase predominates from other causes of intrahepatic cholestasis.

Nevertheless, the history (including ingestion of drugs), physical examination and laboratory tests enable a correct diagnosis to be made in 95% of cases (Huete-Armijo and Exton-Smith, 1962).

Laboratory investigations

The usual laboratory tests are employed in investigation of jaundice in old age although invasive techniques should preferably be avoided.

Briefly the tests are as follows:

1. Urine biochemistry

The presence of bilirubin in the urine indicates obstructive jaundice. Absence of urobilinogen occurs in complete biliary obstruction and an increase in urobilinogen in haemolysis and hepatocellular damage.

2. Liver function tests

There are two main groups: (i) excretion of bromsulphthalein and (ii) liver enzymes and flocculation tests. The normal bromsulphthalein retention at 30 min is less than 10%, although after the age of 60 the retention can be up to 15% in healthy individuals; retention of more than 15% should be regarded as indicative of impaired excretion. The serum alkaline phosphatase has a normal range of 21 to 93 U/l (3–13 King–Armstrong (KA) units/100 ml). In obstructive jaundice (both intrahepatic and extrahepatic) it is above 210 U/l (30 KA units). Since some metabolic bone diseases lead to an increase in alkaline phosphatase, estimations of 5-nucleotidase levels should be made in doubtful cases; these are not elevated in bone disease. Gamma-glutamyl transferase is elevated in alcoholic liver disease, and also in metastatic infiltrations of the liver and in cholestasis. Assay of serum bile acids is becoming increasingly available and is a sensitive test to detect mild hepatic damage and to monitor progress in patients with hepatocellular jaundice.

3. Radiography

A plain abdominal X-ray may disclose gall-stones; but since they are very common in old age they may be a coincidental finding. Moreover the absence of shadows does not exclude gall-stones since they are often translucent. Oral cholecystography cannot be carried out in the presence of jaundice, and intravenous cholangiography should be performed only if the serum bilirubin is less than 35 μ mol/l. Endoscopic retrograde cholangio-pancreatography has recently been introduced. Contrast medium is injected into the common bile duct after cannulation of the ampulla of Vater by means of a fibre-optic panendoscope. It is usually a safe and well-tolerated procedure in the elderly and it can establish the presence of biliary or pancreatic disease which might not otherwise be diagnosed except at laparotomy. Barium studies may reveal oesophageal varices and sometimes a distorted duodenum in carcinoma of the head of the pancreas or in carcinoma of the ampulla.

4. Liver biopsy
Using a Menghini needle this procedure is relatively safe, although it should not be carried out if obstructive jaundice, secondary carcinoma or cholangitis are suspected. It is of value in the diagnosis of liver disease.

5. Radio-isotope scanning
The synthetic isotope, technetium (^{99m} Tc) is most often used since it has a short half-life and emits high-energy gamma-rays. Best results are obtained in neoplastic involvement of the liver; the deposits fail to take up the isotope and show as filling defects on the scan.

Management
When the jaundice is obstructive in nature treatment is most likely to be successful if the underlying cause is an impacted gall-stone. Although the mortality of gall-bladder surgery is comparatively high, operative intervention is usually indicated in a patient who has had one or more attacks of jaundice. If the stones are of the cholesterol type and are not calcified they can sometimes be dissolved by the administration of bile salts (chenodeoxycholic acid); treatment must usually be continued for about 6 months. Surgical procedures are of limited value in neoplastic obstructive jaundice. Although a cholecystoenterostomy may cause the jaundice to disappear, life is not appreciably prolonged.

DIVERTICULAR DISEASE OF THE COLON

Diverticular disease of the colon is a major cause of disability in the elderly. The disorder arises from an increase in the pressure gradient between the colonic lumen and the peritoneal cavity causing mucosal herniations at the sites of perforating vessels. Ninety per cent of the diverticula are in the sigmoid region. Manousos and his colleagues (1967) carried out barium studies in unselected outpatients attending all clinics at the Radcliffe Infirmary, Oxford, and found that the prevalence rose from 18.5% in the age group 40–59 years, to 29.2% in age group 60–79, and to 42.1% in those over the age of 80.

Aetiology

Painter and Burkitt (1971) have drawn attention to the striking differences in geographical distribution of this disease; it is the commonest affliction of the colon in Western Europe and North America, but it is extremely rare in Africa, India, China and Korea. They postulate that the high prevalence in Westernized countries is due to dietary fibre deficiency and the high consumption of refined foods. Painter (1969) has shown that a high-residue diet decreases the likelihood of colon diverticula forming, either by preventing the complete closure of the circular muscular fibres or by the sigmoid colon acting as a functional sphincter above the rectum by the action of its circular muscle bands. With a low-residue diet, on the other hand, this effect is produced only by greatly enhanced action of the muscles which become hypertrophied and lead to increased intraluminal pressure and diverticula formation.

Clinical features

In a series of 521 patients presenting with diverticular disease at hospital Parks (1969) found that the main clinical manifestations were: pain in 78% (usually in the lower abdomen, but also in other areas), constipation in 35%, diarrhoea in 19%, alternating constipation and diarrhoea in 9%, rectal bleeding in 30%, a palpable mass in the left iliac fossa in 20%, nausea and vomiting in 20% and urinary symptoms in 13%. Diverticular disease is commonly associated with cholelithiasis and hiatus hernia (Saint's triad). Complications of diverticular disease include intestinal obstruction due to fibrosis and annular constriction of the bowel, perforation with peritonitis, abscess formation and the development of fistulae into the bladder or vagina.

Management

The majority of uncomplicated cases respond to medical treatment by the addition of bran to increase the residue of the diet. According to Painter and his colleagues (1972) this measure promotes symptomatic relief in 85% of cases. Anti-bacterial therapy may be required using neomycin, phthalyl sulphathiazole or septrin (trimethoprim and sulphamethoxazole). Surgical treatment is usually needed when complications develop.

CONSTIPATION

Constipation is the commonest disorder of the gastrointestinal tract in old age. It can be defined as the passage of unduly hard and dry faecal matter. The original definition of Hurst (1937) as a condition in which the residue of food ingested during one day is not excreted within the next 48 hours is unsatisfactory. Since the transit time is usually as long as 3 days even in active old people (and much longer in the confused and bedridden) they would not necessarily complain of constipation. The important factor governing transit time is the composition of the diet and its fibre content. Surveys of the elderly population show that about one-quarter suffer from constipation but rather more than half take laxatives frequently or regularly. The causes and management of constipation in old age have been reviewed by Exton-Smith (1972).

Aetiology

The important *primary* causes are increased gastrointestinal transit time in old age (especially in the physically inactive), overloading of the rectum with incomplete evacuation, diminished awareness of

183

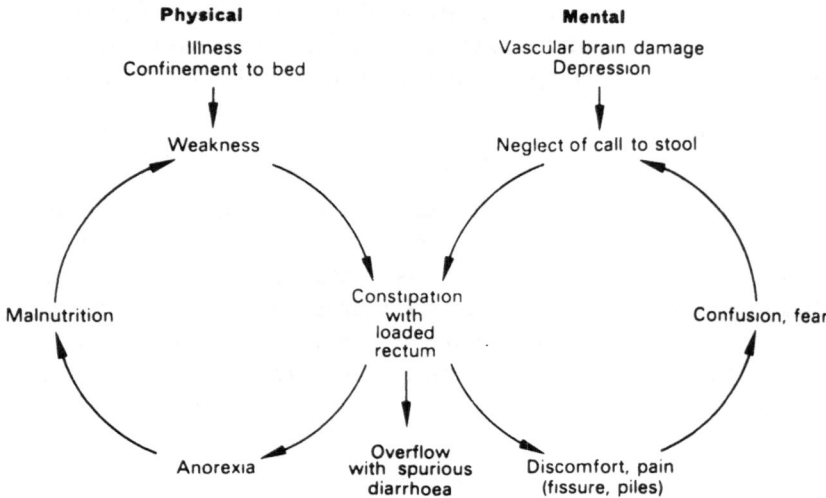

Physical
Illness
Confinement to bed

Weakness

Malnutrition

Anorexia

Constipation with loaded rectum

Overflow with spurious diarrhoea

Mental
Vascular brain damage
Depression

Neglect of call to stool

Confusion, fear

Discomfort, pain (fissure, piles)

Figure 2   Vicious circles of constipation in the elderly (Wilkins, 1968)

rectal distension and the neglect of call to stool. Contributing factors are a faulty diet with insufficient bulk-producing foodstuffs and diminished fluid intake sometimes resulting from fear of urinary incontinence. The main *secondary* causes are the effects of drugs (analgesics, morphine and codeine; salts of iron, calcium and aluminium; ganglion-blocking and anticholinergic drugs), myxoedema, carcinoma and diverticular disease of the colon, anal fissures and haemorrhoids, and psychiatric disorders especially confusional states and depression.

Wilkins (1968) has described the interrelationships between physical and mental factors; the vicious circles which may develop are shown in Figure 2.

Complications

There are several complications which are more prone to occur in the elderly. Straining at stool leads to changes in coronary and cerebral circulations; cases of sudden death have been reported in patients with organic heart disease and syncope can occur as the result of reduction in cerebral blood flow. In the gastrointestinal tract the symptoms of hiatus hernia may be aggravated by constipation, mega-colon may develop as the result of atony of the bowel musculature and when the sigmoid colon is affected volvulus with intestinal obstruction may occur. The commonest sequel of constipation in old age is the development of faecal impaction.

Faecal impaction

Faecal impaction is a more common sequel of constipation in the elderly than in other age groups. The underlying mechanism is slowing of the passage of bowel contents and the excessive absorption of fluids. The hardened faeces are moulded by movements of the bowel and lubricated by excess mucus secretion. Owing to lack of awareness of rectal distension the scybalae remain *in situ* and become smooth and rounded in appearance, even resembling gall-stones. In 98% of cases the impaction is in the rectum, but rarely it can occur at other sites in the ascending, transverse and descending colon.

There are five main ways in which faecal impaction may present:

1. Faecal incontinence
The impacted faeces act as a ball-valve obstruction in the rectum; the stools above the obstruction become liquefied by bacterial action and are passed as *spurious* diarrhoea. Incontinence persists owing to the stretching of the anal ring.

2. Intestinal obstruction
As in other causes of obstruction the features may be gross distension of the abdomen, vomiting, dehydration and the appearance of fluid levels on the abdominal radiograph. Unless the cause of obstruction is recognized by rectal examination the patient may be subjected to unnecessary surgical intervention.

3. Mental disturbances
Not only is the patient with a chronic confusional state more likely to develop faecal impaction, but this in turn is liable to aggravate confusion and to cause restlessness and noisy behaviour; thus a vicious circle is established. Treatment of the impaction often leads to

185

marked improvement, whereas prescription of tranquillizers without attention to the underlying cause will only aggravate the condition.

4. Rectal haemorrhage
Ulceration of the bowel wall with bleeding can occur, but it is essential to exclude rectal neoplasm before it is assumed that haemorrhage is due to this cause.

5. Urinary retention
Pressure on the bladder neck from the distended rectum can cause urinary incontinence with or without overflow incontinence.

Management of constipation
The majority of cases of constipation are primary in origin but treatment should only be started when this has been established and secondary causes of constipation have been excluded as far as possible. The patient should be reassured that regular bowel action can be achieved with appropriate treatment. Physical activity must be encouraged and the patient induced to take adequate fluids. A low-residue diet should be supplemented by additional dietary fibre often best given in the form of bran. Drugs known to cause constipation should as far as possible be avoided. Before laxatives are given, and before the diet is supplemented with fibre, faecal impaction must be treated either with suppositories or enemata (repeated if necessary) and in some cases by manual removal of the faeces after digital fragmentation of the mass.

Strong purgatives must be avoided since many of them act on the small intestine and produce watery stools. The laxative of choice is one which stimulates gut smooth muscle activity, has a selective action on the large bowel, and is substantially free from adverse effects. Good results with the restoration of regular bowel habits can often be achieved with standardized senna (Senokot), even in elderly patients with chronic brain syndromes. In every case there must be careful adjustment of the dosage according to the needs of the individual patient. The dose may vary from two tablets per day to four tablets given twice a day. A combination of a laxative and a colloidal agent such as Fibogel may allow the dosage of the laxative to be reduced. Bisacodyl also acts by stimulating peristalsis in the colon. It can be given orally or as a suppository. In the latter form it is more effective than glycerine suppositories. Enemata, which are normally required in the initial treatment of severe constipation and faecal impaction, are best given in small volume disposable form (e.g. Fletcher's enema which contains sodium phosphate and diphosphate in a 120 ml plastic container).

Therapeutic hazards from the use of laxatives

In the elderly the ill effects of abuse of laxatives are common and are often greater than those of constipation. They include:

Dehydration and electrolyte disturbances
These result from the outpouring of large amounts of fluid into the lumen of the bowel. Great weakness and apathy are common complaints, but the real danger lies in impairment of homeostasis in old age with a diminished ability to tolerate changes in circulatory blood volume.

Hypokalaemia
This is sometimes of severe degree, especially following the use of irritant purgatives. Occasionally it leads to muscular paralysis. There is also an increased danger of digitalis intoxication in patients being treated for congestive cardiac failure.

Hypermagnesiumaemia
This condition can occur especially in the presence of renal impairment when magnesium sulphate is used as a laxative.

Intestinal obstruction
This has been reported following the use of hydrophilic colloids when the expanded mass blocks the gut lumen.

Perforation of the bowel
Perforation may occur when a laxative is given in the presence of an inflammatory lesion.

187

Impaired absorption of vitamin D
This condition, and the development of osteomalacia, can occur from the continued use of liquid paraffin.

Lipoid pneumonia
This is a special hazard associated with liquid paraffin. After taking the oil at night small amounts may remain in the mouth and pharynx and are aspirated during sleep. The oil accumulates in the bronchioles and causes inflammation and fibrosis. The danger of aspiration is greatest when pharyngeal movements are incoordinated following a stroke or in pseudobulbar palsy. So great is the risk of these and other hazards due to liquid paraffin that it should now no longer be used as a laxative.

DIARRHOEA

Diarrhoea is a common disorder in the elderly which can give rise to diagnostic difficulties. In some cases it is trivial due to dietary indiscretions, whilst in others it is a manifestation of serious disease both within and outside the alimentary system.

Causes

Some important causes in the elderly are shown below:

Gastrointestinal	*Metabolic*
Carcinoma of colon	Uraemia
Diverticular disease	Diabetes
Faecal impaction with 'spurious' diarrhoea	Thyrotoxicosis
Ischaemic colitis	*Iatrogenic*
Ulcerative colitis	Abuse of purgatives
Bacillary dysentery	Broad spectrum antibiotics
Malabsorption syndromes	Digoxin toxicity

Alimentary system

Diagnosis

A careful history is necessary to ascertain the nature of the bowel disturbance and associated symptoms, together with an enquiry into the use of purgatives and other drugs. Physical examination may reveal an abdominal mass in carcinoma of the colon and in diverticular disease and the scybalae of faecal impaction. In patients with diabetes there may be other signs of autonomic neuropathy producing the 'nocturnal diarrhoea of elderly diabetics'. A positive occult blood test is found in patients with carcinoma, ischaemic colitis, ulcerative colitis and often in diverticular disease. In these cases barium examination and colonoscopy are essential for accurate diagnosis. Bacteriological investigations should be carried out in suspected cases of dysentery.

Management

When an infective cause is found, a course of non-absorbable antibiotic such as neomycin or phthalyl sulphathiazole should be prescribed. Symptomatic treatment of diarrhoea with agents which reduce intestinal motility, such as codeine phosphate, is sometimes successful in reducing the frequency of bowel movements. The main danger of severe or prolonged diarrhoea in the elderly is the occurrence of dehydration and electrolyte disturbances which are badly tolerated owing to failing capacity for homeostasis. Reduction in circulatory blood volume and electrolyte abnormalities must be quickly corrected.

FAECAL INCONTINENCE

In geriatric practice faecal incontinence is second in importance to urinary incontinence as a major problem of medical and nursing care. In a survey of 2223 elderly hospital patients Brocklehurst (1951) found that 312 were incontinent; of this total 25% were incontinent of urine only, 72% were incontinent of urine and faeces, and only 3% were incontinent of faeces alone.

Aetiology

There are three main causes of faecal incontinence in old age.

1. Neurogenic

The disorder responsible for faecal incontinence is analogous to that occurring in the uninhibited neurogenic bladder causing urinary incontinence. In the normal process of defaecation the faecal mass moves from the descending colon into the rectum when a gastrocolic reflex is produced by the ingestion of food. The consequent distension of the rectum causes rectal contractions and relaxation of the internal sphincter. In the normal individual defaecation can be postponed voluntarily by inhibition of contractions and the rapid restoration of tone in the internal sphincter. In the elderly patient suffering from neurogenic faecal incontinence voluntary control is impaired or lost. The impairment of voluntary control is particularly marked in senile (Alzheimer type) and in multi-infarct dementia.

2. 'Spurious' diarrhoea

In patients with faecal impaction (see page 185) liquefaction of faeces occurs above the ball-valve obstruction and these are passed as 'spurious' diarrhoea.

3. Symptomatic

In patients suffering from diarrhoea (see page 188) the voluntary control mechanisms may be ineffective in preventing the passage of liquid faeces from the rectum.

Management

The correct management of faecal incontinence depends upon making an accurate diagnosis of the underlying cause. In this respect it is important to exclude organic disease of the colon and rectum and other causes of diarrhoea. Rectal examination may reveal faecal impaction and this should be treated accordingly. If the rectum is empty sigmoidoscopy and barium enema examination should be carried out. Any local lesions should be treated if possible. Neurogenic incontinence should be managed by inducing constipation and alternated with planned evacuation of the bowel. Jarrett and Exton-Smith (1960) have described a regimen in which kaolin and morphine are given in the morning and standardized senna (Senokot) in the evening. Brocklehurst (1972) recommends giving a constipating drug for a longer period and a planned evacuation is obtained on the 5th–7th day by the use of enemata or suppositories.

REFERENCES

Andrews, J., Letcher, M. and Brook, M. (1969). Vitamin C supplementation in the elderly. A 17-month trial in an old people's home. *Br. Med. J.*, **2,** 416
Brocklehurst, J. C. (1951). In *Incontinence in Old People*. (Edinburgh Livingstone)
Brocklehurst, J. C. (1972). Bowel management in the neurologically disabled. The problems in old age. *Proc. R. Soc. Med.*, **65,** 66
Dent, C. E., Stokes, J. F. and Carpenter, M. E. (1961). Death from hypothermia in steatorrhoea. *Lancet*, **i,** 748
Dudley, F. J., Scheuer, P. J. and Sherlock, S. (1972). Natural history of hepatitis-associated antigen-positive chronic liver disease. *Lancet*, **ii,** 1388
Exton-Smith, A. N. (1972). Constipation in geriatrics. In F. Avery Jones and E. W. Godding (eds). *Management of Constipation*. (Oxford: Blackwell)
Exton-Smith, A. N. and Osborne, G. (1961). Barium studies in the aged. *Br. Med. J.*, **1,** 1799
Huete-Armijo, A. and Exton-Smith, A. N. (1962). Causes and diagnosis of jaundice in the elderly. *Br. Med. J.*, **1,** 1113
Hurst, A. F. (1937). Constipation. In H. Rolleston (eds.). *British Encyclopaedia of Medical Practice*. (London: Butterworth)
Jarrett, A. S. and Exton-Smith, A. N. (1960). Treatment of faecal incontinence. Lancet, **i,** 925
Kendall, M. J. (1970). The influence of age on the xylose absorption test. *Gut*, **11,** 498

191

Manousos, O. N., Truelove, S. C. and Lumsden, K. (1967). Transit times of food in patients with diverticulosis or irritable colon syndrome and normal subjects. *Br. Med. J.*, **3,** 760

Painter, N. S. (1969). Diverticular disease of the colon: the disease of the century. *Lancet*, **ii,** 586

Painter, N. S. and Burkitt, D. P. (1971). Diverticular disease of the colon, a deficiency disease of western civilisation. *Br. Med. J.*, **2,** 450

Painter, N. S., Almeida, A. S. and Colebourne, K. W. (1972). Unprocessed bran in treatment of diverticular disease of the colon. *Br. Med. J.*, **2,** 137

Parks, T. G. (1969). Natural history of diverticular disease of the colon. *Br. Med. J.*, **4,** 639

Price, H. L., Gassard, B. G. and Dawson, A. M. (1977). Steatorrhoea in the elderly. *Br. Med. J.*, **1,** 1582

Shorter, R. G., Paton, A. and Pinniger, J. L. (1959). Hepatic jaundice. *Q. J. Med.*, **28,** 43

Strange, S. L. (1963). Giant innocent gastric ulcer in the elderly. *Gerontol. Clin.*, **5,** 171

Wilkins, E. G. (1968). Constipation in the elderly. *Postgrad. Med. J.*, **44,** 728

9
Nutrition

Changes in nutritional status of elderly people are brought about by alterations in their socio-economic circumstances, which often occur about the time of retirement, and by the increasing incidence of disease and disability which lead to changes in dietary intake, absorption and metabolism of nutrients. The effects of disease and disabilities become more marked during the second half of the eighth decade. Thus, although frank malnutrition has been largely eliminated from most sections of our population, it is still found amongst the elderly as a consequence of the operation of these factors.

AGEING AND NUTRITION

Rate of ageing

The first experimental proof that restriction of food intake can influence life span of animals came with the work of McCay and his colleagues (1935) who showed that rats whose growth was almost completely arrested by a period of severe food restriction lived longer than those fed *ad-libitum*. According to Miller and Payne (1968) when experiments have been repeated most observers have commented upon the miserable state of the long-living rats; they are seen

193

to be underweight and in poor condition. These authors examined the longevity of animals whose nutrient intake was adjusted to growth rather than being fed with a dietary regime of constant composition throughout life. Five different regimes were used and the greatest prolongation of life was achieved in animals fed a stock diet until mature (120 days) and thereafter a mixture of 20% stock diet and 80% starch. Compared with animals on a stock diet throughout life these animals had a maximum life span 100 days longer and their mean life expectancy was 28% longer; moreover, they appeared healthy in old age. This extended life span after maturity must be contrasted with the rats in the McCay experiments in which there is an extended juvenile life.

Ross and Bras (1974) have shown that the frequency of various types of tumour and several age-related diseases can be modified by dietary means. The rats under investigation were allowed a choice of three complete balanced diets differing only in the amounts of sugar and protein they contained; in this self-selection method (S-S) each rat could eat as much or as little as it liked of each kind of food. As a control, three other groups of rats were fed on low, intermediate and high protein diets. The rats on the S-S regime grew more quickly than the others and reached higher body weights, but they had a far higher incidence of tumours and of renal, cardiac and prostate gland diseases. Two-thirds of the S-S rats had three or more diseases at the time of death, while of the rats fed low, intermediate or high protein diets alone, only 9, 26 and 28% respectively had multiple affections at the time of death. These diseases have certain similarities in rat and man and occupy comparable positions in the life spans of the two species. In brief, the results of animal experiments indicate that overfeeding in earlier life hastens maturity and shortens life, and overfeeding after maturity shortens life and increases the incidence of certain diseases in old age.

Metabolic rate

The total energy production per square metre of body surface area falls progressively with advancing age; the average decrement is about 12 cal/m^2 per hour between the ages of 20 and 90 years. The fall is believed to be due to a loss of metabolizing tissues with age since animal experiments show that there is no decrease in oxygen uptake of tissue slices, homogenates or isolated mitochondria from rat heart, liver and kidney. This total energy production per 24 hours is the sum of basal energy production and that required for daily activities. There is evidence that the calories required for activities fall more than the basal calories, especially in very old individuals. Thus the reduction in energy metabolism of older subjects is a reflection of tissue loss and to a greater extent the reduction in physical activity which becomes especially pronounced after the age of 75. The considerable differences in energy expenditure observed in very old people can often be accounted for by such causes as degenerative joint disease and disorders of the respiratory and cardiovascular systems.

TABLE 1

RECOMMENDED DAILY INTAKES OF ENERGY AND NUTRIENTS FOR ELDERLY PEOPLE IN THE UK (FROM DHSS REPORT 1969)

	Men		Women	
	65–74	75 and over	55–74	75 and over
Energy (cal)	2350	2100	2050	1900
(MJ)	9.8	8.8	8.6	8.0
Protein (g)	59	53	51	48
Calcium (mg)	500	500	500	500
Iron (mg)	10	10	10	10
Thiamine (mg)	0.9	0.8	0.8	0.7
Riboflavine (mg)	1.7	1.7	1.3	1.3
Nicotinic acid (mg)	18	18	15	15
Ascorbic acid (mg)	30	30	30	30
Vitamin A (μg retinol equiv.)	750	750	750	750
Vitamin D (μg cholecalciferol)	2.5	2.5	2.5	2.5

Recommended intake of nutrients

Many countries have produced recommendations for daily intakes of energy and nutrients. The values for old people recommended by the Department of Health and Social Security (1969) are summarized in Table 1. These recommendations for the elderly are based on estimates of the average rate at which activities decline; that is, they take account of the diminution in energy expenditure associated with the increasing incidence of physical infirmity with age. Nevertheless, there are many individuals whose activities are well maintained in old age and whose calorie intakes are much greater than the recommended values.

MALNUTRITION

Malnutrition may be defined as a disturbance of form or function due to lack of (or excess of) calories or of one or more nutrients (DHSS, 1972). Thus both obesity and undernutrition are included in this definition. Obesity can be a problem in old age and after the age of 75 it is much more common in women than in men, but it usually results from long-standing faulty eating habits, often accentuated in old age by a reduction in physical activity. Undernutrition, on the other hand, results from both environmental and physical factors affecting people in later life.

There are two main groups of factors that lead to nutritional deficiency in the elderly (Exton-Smith, 1971) and these are summarized in Table 2.

Ignorance

The King Edward's Hospital Fund Survey (Exton-Smith and Stanton, 1965) showed that ignorance of the basic facts of nutrition is prevalent in elderly women. Their views had usually been formulated many years ago, and even in childhood, when dietary habits had often been dictated by financial stringency. It is likely that in men ignorance is even more important: for example, a man who is recently widowed may have to fend for himself for the first time and he may have little idea of what constitutes a balanced diet. Widower's scurvy is seen most often in the man living alone eating mostly packaged food, tea, bread, butter and jam.

TABLE 2
CAUSES OF NUTRITIONAL DEFICIENCIES

Primary	Secondary
Ignorance	Impaired appetite
Social isolation	Masticatory inefficiency
Physical disability	Malabsorption
Mental disturbance	Alcoholism
Iatrogenic	Drugs
Poverty	Increased requirements

Social isolation

Several studies have shown that dietary intake is related to the number of outside interests of old people. It is usually better in those old people who eat at clubs in the company of others. By contrast, for many old people living alone in social isolation there is loss of interest sometimes amounting to apathy and consequent neglect in the preparation of food. What food is usually eaten is taken in the form of snacks.

Physical disabilities

Elderly people with physical disorders such as hemiplegia, arthritis and impairment of vision may have difficulty in getting and preparing food. This applies particularly to the housebound living alone without adequate support from others.

Mental disturbances

The unmet medical, nursing and social needs of the elderly are greatest in those with psychiatric disorders. Malnutrition also occurs in this group which consists mainly of old people suffering from chronic brain syndrome and confusional states. Perhaps even more important is the association between malnutrition and depressive illness, which leads to a disinclination to obtain, to cook and even, in severe cases, to eat food.

Iatrogenic

A badly planned dietary regime may lead to malnutrition, especially when it is continued longer than necessary. Thus cases of scurvy have been reported in patients having a 'gastric' diet for peptic ulcer since this is often deficient in vitamin C.

Poverty

The food eaten by pensioners is often dull, monotonous and tasteless. Old people who are able to supplement their income from savings or from part-time earnings usually have a better diet than those whose sole financial means is the old age pension. In the winter months many old people must make a choice between spending money on food or fuel. Thus poverty is a factor to be considered in the elderly more often than in other age groups.

Impairment of appetite

Both transitory and long-continued impairment of appetite is common in old age. The time taken for recovery of appetite following an infectious illness is longer than in a younger person; frank malnutrition may be precipitated in a person whose nutrition was previously only marginally adequate.

Masticatory inefficiency

A poor state of dentition, and especially ill-fitting dentures, often lead an elderly individual to select soft foods consisting mainly of carbohydrate; the more nutritious foods requiring mastication are avoided.

Old people with few teeth remaining, but no dentures, often perform surprisingly well; often better than those wearing dentures of indifferent quality.

Malabsorption

Mild degrees of malabsorption are not uncommon in the elderly. This may be due to small bowel ischaemia, gluten sensitivity and other causes. The absorption of fat and fat-soluble vitamins and of folic acid and vitamin B_{12} is mainly affected.

Alcohol and drugs

When alcohol intake is excessive, calorie needs may be derived mainly from this source and the intake of other nutrients may be curtailed. Folic acid metabolism is impaired in some alcoholics and megaloblastic anaemia can occur; it is also impaired in those taking barbiturates and anticonvulsant drugs, and in those receiving cytotoxic agents such as methotrexate. Enzyme induction by anticonvulsant drugs can also lead to vitamin D deficiency.

Increased requirements

Negative nitrogen balance and the breakdown of tissue protein can occur in patients who are immobilized in bed for long periods, in those who suffer from long-continued pyrexia and as a result of extensive bedsores with loss of protein-rich fluid.

CLINICAL NUTRITIONAL DEFICIENCIES

The most comprehensive study of the nutritional status of the elderly population so far undertaken was that organized by the Department of Health and Social Security (1972), 'A Nutritional Survey of the Elderly'. Excluding obesity, 27 of the 879 (3%) subjects over the age of 65 participating in the survey were diagnosed by the clinicians as malnourished. The nutritional deficiencies which are to be found in old people will be described and reference will be made to the findings of this Report.

Protein–calorie malnutrition

The total amount of protein in the body declines with age. Forbes and Reina (1970) studied the body composition of subjects at different ages between 25 and 75 years on a longitudinal basis. Using ^{40}K counting it was found that the lean body mass (LBM) declines progressively after the age of 25, whereas fat increases, so that the total body weight fails to reveal the continuous decrease in LBM. Men weighing approximately 75 kg at the age of 25 years have an average LBM of 61 kg and a fat content of 13 kg; at the age of 65 years, however, the LBM has declined by 12 kg (20%), and the body fat has risen by 15 kg (120%), without any marked change in total body weight. Although decline in LBM is continuous after the age of 25, the rate of loss is not constant and it appears to accelerate in old age.

The DHSS recommendations (1969) for *minimum* protein requirements are 39 g and 38 g for men aged 65–75 years and over 75 years respectively, and 36 g and 34 g for women in the corresponding age groups. The actual recommended intakes (59 g, 53 g, 51 g and 48 g respectively) are, however, considerably higher and are calculated on the basis that protein intake should provide 10% of the energy requirements. For the normal utilization of dietary protein sufficient energy must be available, and the protein–energy relationship is more important than the absolute amount of protein.

Serum albumin concentration decreases with advancing age and the total albumin pool is about 20% lower in the elderly subjects compared with the young. Since homeostasis of serum albumin levels in healthy individuals is maintained by a mechanism in the liver which is sensitive to osmotic pressure it is possible that the decrease in serum albumin with age is due to a decline in the sensitivity of this mechanism. In the DHSS Survey of the Elderly (1972), a slight but consistent relationship was found between intake of protein and the bulk of arm muscle (as measured by the arm circumference minus a value for surface fat based on the triceps skinfold thickness). This could partly be explained by larger individuals eating more food and hence more protein. But a part of the relationship was also due to the percentage of energy derived from protein, and this raised the possibility of a relationship between reserves of protein stored in muscle and protein intake as opposed to energy intake.

No consistent relationship was found between protein intake and serum albumin levels, but there was a significant relationship between serum albumin levels and oedema. Serum albumin was less than 3.5 g/100 ml in 48 subjects and 40% had oedema; 22% had oedema when the albumin was 3.5–4.49 g/100 ml and 13% when it was above 4.5 g/100 ml. It is considered that a possible explanation lies in the effects of stress; in this case the stress is non-nutritional disease (mainly cardiac failure) superimposed upon levels of serum albumin which in most cases would have been unassociated with oedema had it not been for the additional burden. Three of the 48 subjects with serum albumin levels of less than 3.5 g/100 ml were thought to have oedema due to protein deficiency; in the remainder, diseases such as congestive cardiac failure imposed a stress on already impaired homeostatic mechanisms. Since the stress could be diagnosed clinically and tended to mask the underlying protein deficiency it was concluded that a state of subclinical nutritional deficiency existed in many of these subjects.

Iron deficiency

The main clinical manifestation of iron deficiency is anaemia (the clinical features are described in Chapter 12). In addition there are other tissue changes such as koilonychia or spoon-shaped deformity of the nails, a smooth and red tongue due to atrophy of the papillae, and rarely a post-cricoid web (Plummer–Vinson syndrome) leading to difficulty in swallowing. Severe anaemia with typical manifestations is rarely due to poor dietary intake of iron alone; in such cases there is nearly always occult or overt gastrointestinal haemorrhage. Nevertheless, nutritional surveys show that dietary lack of iron is common in the elderly population and is related to socio-economic factors.

In the Nutritional Survey of the Elderly (DHSS, 1972) the overall frequency of anaemia was 7.3% and was about the same in the two sexes. A significant correlation was found between Hb level and mode of living. When all persons were grouped together 9% of those living alone had anaemia compared with 6% of those who lived with a spouse or relative ($p < 0.01$). In addition there was a significant correlation between the Hb concentration and serum iron (SI) level. Overt iron deficiency as measured by an SI of less than 60μ g/100 ml and a total iron binding capacity (TIBC) higher than 400 μ g/100 ml was found in 4.7% of elderly men and 13.2% of elderly women. The most likely explanation of this difference is the lower iron intake of most groups of elderly women; thus in six areas surveyed in only one group of women (the 65–74 age group in Angus) was the mean intake of iron greater than the recommended intake of 10 mg/day, whereas by contrast only one group of men (75+ age group in Sunderland) failed to reach the recommended intake. It is of interest that in anaemic subjects, iron deficiency was the sole cause of anaemia in only 12.9%. Iron deficiency was more often associated with sub-normal levels of serum folate or of vitamin B_{12}; in 20% of anaemic subjects all three serum levels were abnormal.

Riboflavin deficiency

Changes in the mucous membranes of the tongue and lips due to riboflavin deficiency include:

cheilosis – red, denuded often scaly epithelium at the line of closure of the lips;
angular stomatitis – greyish-white sodden and swollen epithelium progressing to fissure at the angles of the mouth;
naso-labial seborrhoea – enlarged follicles around the sides of the nose and plugged with sebaceous material;
glossitis – bare, red, smooth tongue with loss of filiform papillae, sometimes associated with fissuring and enlargement of the fungiform papillae.

These changes are characteristically found in riboflavin deficiency, but some of them may be related to deficiency of nicotinamide, possibly pyridoxine. There is a conflict of opinion on the extent to which these changes can be reversed by vitamin supplementation.

The clinical manifestations of other B group vitamins are mainly in the nervous system.

Thiamine deficiency

Deficiency of thiamine can cause peripheral neuropathy and is usually associated with alcoholism. Response to thiamine administration is variable and in some cases the neuropathy persists due to irreversible neurological damage. Another important manifestation of thiamine deficiency is Wernicke's encephalopathy due to petechial haemorrhages in the mid-brain particularly in the region of the mamillary bodies. The clinical features include ophthalmoplegia, postural hypotension, intellectual impairment and memory disturbances (Korsakoff's psychosis). Hypothermia occurs in some cases and is probably due to involvement of the autonomic nervous system; The nutritional status of many old people admitted to hospital with accidental hypothermia is often unsatisfactory. The memory disturbance in patients with Wernicke's encephalopathy is usually dramatically improved by massive doses of thiamine. The extent to which a relative thiamine deficiency associated with toxic infective processes can lead to mental confusion in the absence of signs of Wernicke's disease needs further investigation.

Nicotinamide deficiency

Deficiency of nicotinamide causes pellagra, a disease which is characterized by three Ds – dermatitis, diarrhoea and dementia. Other neurological manifestations besides dementia include peripheral neuropathy, myelopathy and amblyopia. Like thiamine deficiency, the manifestations of nicotinamide deficiency are usually found in chronic alcoholics and patients suffering from acute illnesses particularly associated with vomiting (carcinoma of the stomach, pancreas, colon and intestinal obstruction).

Folate deficiency

The manifestations include megaloblastic anaemia (see Chapter 12), glossitis, peripheral neuropathy and mental changes (confusion, depression, apathy and intellectual impairment). The main causes in the elderly are inadequate intake, malabsorption, increased utilization and impaired effectiveness. A mixed diet contains 500–800 mg folate per day, but folate in the reduced form is readily destroyed by sunlight, oxidation and cooking. Dietary deficiency is often associated with mental and physical disabilities which interfere with shopping and cooking. Thus investigations of the folate status of elderly patients in hospital show that it is most likely to be inferior in those with severe disabilities, particularly chronic brain syndrome. Folate requirements are increased when cell turnover increases, e.g. in haemolytic anaemia, myeloproliferative syndromes, carcinoma or some chronic inflammatory conditions. Under certain circumstances the effectiveness of available folate is impaired – in vitamin C deficiency which inhibits folate coenzymes and leads to the megaloblastic anaemia of scurvy, and following the use of such drugs as methotrexate, anticonvulsants, barbiturates and trimethoprim which interfere with folate metabolism.

Ascorbic acid deficiency

Scurvy has almost disappeared from our population, but it occasionally occurs in the elderly, especially in men. The manifestations include swelling and bleeding from the gums (not seen in edentulous individuals), weakness, anaemia, extensive haemorrhages in the skin of legs and arms ('sheet' haemorrhages) and sometimes haemorrhages at other sites. Anaemia is common in scurvy; it is usually normocytic or macrocytic with normoblastic or macronormoblastic erythropoiesis, but cases of true megaloblastic anaemia have been reported. The origin of anaemia is often multifactorial: haemolysis, bleeding, dietary deficiency of iron and derangement of red cell metabolism may each be responsible. Megaloblastic change has been attributed either to an associated dietary folate deficiency or to impairment of folate metabolism in scurvy. Mental disturbances are probably common in scurvy, taking the form of depression and personality changes. Wound healing may be delayed in vitamin C deficiency and the administration of vitamin C may promote the healing of pressure sores by increasing collagen formation.

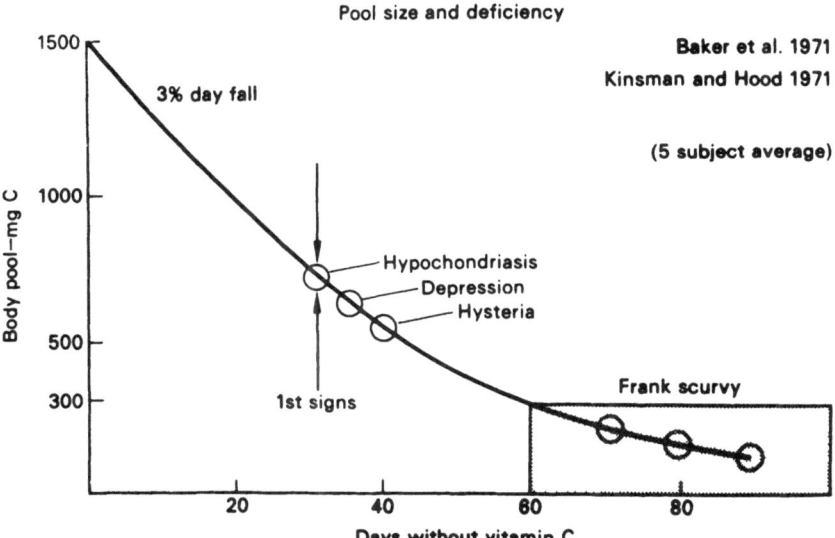

Figure 1 Pool size and deficiency of vitamin C

When the dietary intake of vitamin C is adequate (more than 30 mg/day) the total body store of this vitamin is about 1500 mg. If the intake ceases the body pool size immediately begins to decline at about 3% per day. The times of onset of manifestations are shown in Figure 1. The body stores of vitamin C, as measured by leukocyte ascorbic acid (LAA) are diminished in many old people. LAA levels are lower in the elderly than in younger subjects, lower in winter than in summer, and lower in men than in women. Diminished ascorbic acid levels have been reported in institutionalized old people. They have been attributed to: the effects of cooking in institutions of such foods as potatoes, the delay in delivery of the meal to the recipient, and to an inadequate supply of fruit and fruit juices. Similar factors may be responsible for the inferior vitamin C status of old people receiving meals-on-wheels, mainly the housebound. These meals are cooked in institutions and are kept hot for several hours in containers before they are delivered. Stanton (1971) has shown that 90% of the vitamin C may be destroyed before the meal is served. Davies and others (1973), in a study of a meals-on-wheels service supplied on average 2–3 days per week, have demonstrated that the vitamin C intake may be considerably less on those days on which the old person receives a domiciliary meal compared with days on which he or she cooks the meal at home.

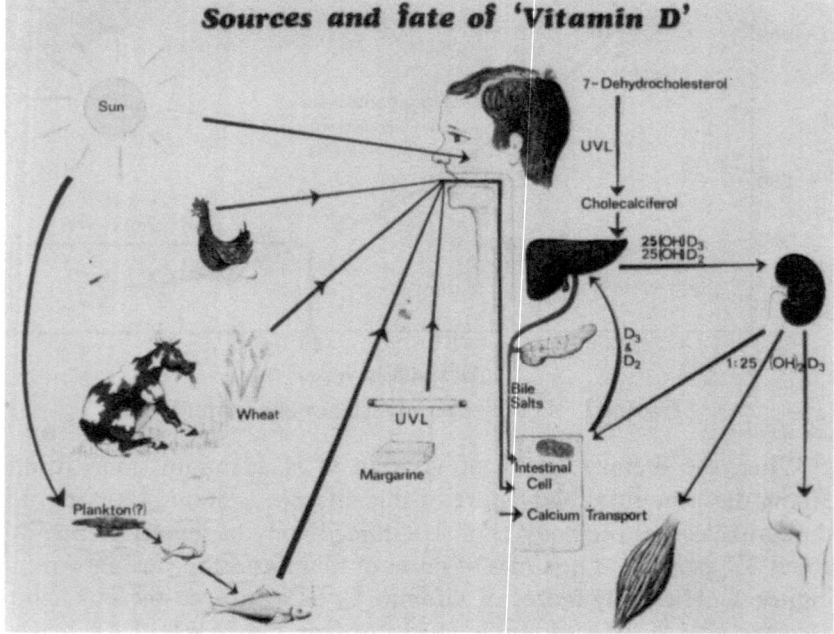

Figure 2 Vitamin D metabolism: sources, transport and function (with kind permission of Dr D. Corless)

Vitamin D deficiency

The sources of vitamin D and its metabolism and utilization are shown in Figure 2. The clinical features of osteomalacia which is caused by vitamin D deficiency are described in Chapter 14. There are many causes in old age and often several factors operate together in the same individual. The importance of some of these factors have been elucidated by measurement of serum levels of 25-hydroxychole-calciferol (25-HCC) in various groups of the population, for example in young active subjects, in the elderly at home, in old people in institutions, in patients with osteomalacia and in patients with femoral neck fracture.

Simple vitamin D lack
This may be due to a low dietary intake of vitamin D or the lack of exposure to sunlight. Stamp and Round (1974) have shown seasonal variations in the serum levels of 25-HCC both in old and young subjects and they conclude that summer sunlight is important, and possibly the chief determinant of vitamin D nutrition in Britain. The 25-HCC levels are lower in old people compared with the young. In this report, housebound old people may be at the greatest disadvantage since they lack exposure to sunlight and often have very low dietary intakes; 48% of housebound women aged 70–79 years had a dietary intake of less than 30 i.u. per day compared with 13% of active women of similar age (Exton-Smith *et al.*, 1972).

Malabsorption
Minor and even more severe degrees of malabsorption are not uncommon in old age. Enteropathy due to rye and wheat gluten sensitivity similar to that causing childhood coeliac disease is still seen in patients in their 70s.

PREVENTION OF MALNUTRITION

The clinical significance of malnutrition is far greater than its incidence might suggest, since in almost every case it is treatable with excellent results. Difficulties in detection of the early signs of malnutrition are similar to those encountered in the early recognition of many diseases in old age. But in the case of nutritional deficiencies there are two further difficulties: for almost every nutrient there is a

207

long latent period before a low intake leads to overt clinical manifestations, and early diagnosis must depend upon the finding of abnormalities in special tests, including biochemical and haematological investigations; secondly, in the elderly the true significance of departures from normality revealed by these tests is unknown. Many of the abnormalities can be related to low intakes of certain nutrients, but in old age there is considerable variation between individuals. Although in younger persons the margin of safety is wide, in old age homeostatic mechanisms are often impaired and the precarious physiological balance may be upset by the operation of medical and environmental hazards to which the elderly are prone. Frank malnutrition may be precipitated by such stress in those individuals whose nutrition is only marginally adequate.

Vulnerable groups

Old people especially at risk are the socially isolated; those with physical disability, including impairment of the special senses which contribute to isolation; the recently bereaved; very old men living alone; and those with mental disorders, particularly depression. Unless these vulnerable groups can be identified preventive measures would have to be applied to all old people irrespective of the fact that the majority will never suffer from malnutrition. The undesirability and the inefficiency of applying such procedures can be overcome only by the recognition of those especially at risk. The application of preventive measures to these smaller groups rather than to the entire elderly population becomes a manageable proposition.

The housebound, who account for 8–10% of old people living in their homes, constitute the largest group at risk. Physical and mental disorder in old age not only affects the mode of living and social relationships of those afflicted, but also the dietary pattern and nutritional status. Since the majority of the housebound are already known to the health and social services, the prevention of malnutrition in this group should present less difficulty than in other vulnerable groups who are not so readily identifiable.

Nutrition

Assessment of nutritional status

When the groups of old people especially at risk have been identified the prevention of malnutrition is the responsibility of the primary medical care team. Although the assessment of dietary intakes should ideally be made by dietitians, their skills are not often available for old people at home. A rough guide to the quality of the diet can be obtained by health visitors using simple scoring systems which are based on the number of main meals and the frequency of consumption of certain foods containing protein (meat, bread, eggs, cheese and milk). If the diet is found to be insufficient means must be sought for improving nutritional intake; this may entail instruction by a dietitian or health visitor either individually or when old people attend clubs or day centres. When clinical malnutrition is suspected the diagnosis can sometimes be confirmed by the general practitioner using appropriate biochemical and haematological investigations; in other instances, however, referral to hospital for more specialized investigations will be necessary; for example, for bone biopsy when there are clinical findings suggestive of osteomalacia.

Club meals and meals-on-wheels

It has been shown that there is often an improvement in nutrient intake when old people eat at clubs in the company of others. Many find that it is more convenient to have a club meal since there is no shopping, cooking or washing-up to be done. The King Edward's Hospital Fund Survey (Exton-Smith and Stanton, 1965) showed that in order to make an effective contribution to the total dietary intake at least four club meals a week should be eaten. The club or domiciliary meal must be as nutritious as possible since the recipient tends to regard it as the main meal of the day and often takes only snacks at other times.

About 2% of old people receive meals-on-wheels, but the real need is probably much greater than this. The meals service is usually provided by the WRVS and the regular visits to the homes of housebound old people do much to prevent social isolation. One of the disadvantages of the present system of delivery is that food must be kept hot

209

for several hours after cooking before the meal reaches the old person's home. During this time at least some of the nutritive value is lost. There is need for experiment in this field. In several areas the provision of frozen meals has been tried. The meal can be cooked immediately before it is eaten and since food is delivered only once a week the service is economical in personnel. The main disadvantages, however, are that there may be no proper facilities for cold storage, the patient may be unable to cook the meal himself and he is visited much less frequently by voluntary workers.

Nutrient supplementation

The most satisfactory means of promoting good nutrition is by improving the quality, and in some cases the quantity, of the diet. Thus for those whose consumption of vitamin C is inadequate, intake could be improved by the addition of oranges, blackcurrant juice, rose hip syrup or tomatoes. The alternative of prescribing ascorbic acid tablets is satisfactory, but less desirable. The very low intake of vitamin D by many old people must lead to consideration of supplementation. A means of increasing the intake would be by the fortification of milk, which is a procedure adopted in the United States. In the first instance the distribution of fortified milk might best be restricted to housebound old people who tend to have the lowest vitamin D intakes and lack of exposure to sunlight.

It is important that supplementation should only be introduced after the results of carefully controlled trials are available to assess the benefits derived from increased intakes. Once the practice of supplementation has become widespread it is difficult to prove the benefits. Moreover there is an understandable reluctance to withdraw a prophylactic measure on the basis of doubts about its value when it has been employed for several years.

REFERENCES

Davies, L., Hastrop, K. and Bender, A. E. (1973). Ascorbic acid in meals-on-wheels. *Mod. Geriat.*, **3,** 390

DHSS (1969) Recommended intakes of nutrients for the United Kingdom. *Report on Public Health and Medical Subjects, No. 120.* (London: HMSO)

DHSS (1972) A nutrition survey of the elderly. *Report on Public Health and Medical Subjects, No. 3.* (London: HMSO)

Exton-Smith, A. N. (1971) Nutrition of the elderly. *Br. J. Hosp. Med.,* **5,** 639

Exton-Smith, A. N. and Stanton, B. R. (1965). *Report on an Investigation into the Dietary of Elderly Women Living Alone.* (London: King Edward's Hospital Fund)

Exton-Smith, A. N., Stanton, B. R. and Windsor, A. C. M. (1972). *Nutrition of housebound old people.* (London: King Edward's Hospital Fund)

Forbes, G. B. and Reina, J. C. (1970). Adult lean body mass declines with age; some longitudinal observations. *Metabolism,* **19,** 653

McCay, C. M., Crowell, M. R. and Maynard, L. A. (1935). Effect of retarded growth upon the length of life span and upon the ultimate body size. *J. Nutr.,* **10,** 63

Miller, D. S. and Payne, P. R. (1968). Longevity and protein intake. *Expl. Gerontol.* **3,** 231

Ross, M. H. and Bras, G. (1974). Dietary preference and disease of age. *Nature,* **250,** 263

Stamp, T. C. B. and Round, J. M. (1974). Seasonal changes in human plasma levels of 25-hydroxyvitamin D. *Nature,* **247,** 563

Stanton, B. R. (1971). *Meals for the Elderly.* (London: King Edward's Hospital Fund)

10
Urogenital system

AGEING

With increasing age the kidney atrophies, affecting the cortex more than the medulla. Interstitial fibrosis is most marked in the medulla with coarse scarring also seen in a small percentage of cases. There are, however, considerable variations in the appearance of the kidney in old age.

The number of glomeruli halve between the fourth and seventh decade and the glomerular and tubular basement membrane thickens. Renal arteriosclerosis is generally considered to be an age-related change and not due to hypertension.

Glomerular and tubular function decrease at the same rate. There is a steady reduction in urine concentrating capacity, transport maximum of glucose, ability to excrete an acid load and renal tubular response to antidiuretic hormone. The fall in glomerular filtration rate (GFR) is linear up to the fifth or sixth decade but becomes much greater thereafter (McLachlan, 1978). Sick old people have a lower GFR than healthy subjects and age alone is not a reliable predictor of GFR (Denham, Hodkinson and Fisher, 1975). Although endogenous creatinine production may be very low in thin elderly people, the serum urea and creatinine levels are determined by GFR and body weight, and are independent of age.

The interpretation of biochemical data has been reviewed by Hodkinson (1978) who found that renal impairment is common in ill old people, as shown by a 95% range for urea of 3.1–20.6 mmol/l (18–124 mg/100 ml). Consequently, serum phosphate results are raised to 0.73–1.70 mmol/l (2.25–5.25 mg/100 ml). Uric acid levels are also raised by renal impairment. Bicarbonate results are negatively correlated and potassium positively correlated with urea. Modest rises in blood urea (10 mmol/l, 60 mg/100 ml) are found even in normal elderly people as a consequence of renal impairment, and should not be a cause for concern.

It is generally agreed that there is a high prevalence of bacteriuria among the elderly and most studies have found that women are more affected than men (Akhtar *et al.*, 1972). Among people living in the community significant bacteriuria (100 000+ organisms/ml) is present in 2–4% of women between the age of 45 and 64 and in 20% of those aged 65 and over. For men the figures are 3% for the age group 65–70 and 20% after 70 (Brocklehurst *et al.*, 1968 and 1972). The prevalence is higher in hospital where about one-third of elderly patients of both sexes have significant bacteriuria.

The high prevalence of bacteriuria in the elderly is probably due to the increasing frequency of a neuropathic bladder which has two effects. First, because of inefficiency of the micturition reflex there is usually residual urine, which favours bacterial growth. Secondly, the high intravesical pressure produced by unstable detrusor contractions can reduce the capillary blood flow to the bladder wall and weaken resistance to infection (Lapides and Costello, 1969). Another possible cause for increased residual urine in elderly women is bladder neck obstruction, a well-recognized but poorly understood condition. In men the reduction of prostatic fluid with its antibacterial action may be a contributory factor, in addition to the effect of bladder outflow obstruction due to prostatic hypertrophy.

Other evidence for the increase of a neuropathic bladder with age is nocturia, which is present in 70% of men and 61% of women over the age of 65. Nocturia is a symptom of cerebral deterioration but it is not associated with incontinence (Brocklehurst *et al.*, 1968).

Asymptomatic urinary tract infections are common in the elderly and some old people have symptoms of dysuria, nocturnal frequency and precipitancy without infection. Chronic urinary tract infections are not a cause of incontinence. The majority of urinary infections in the elderly are confined to the bladder and are not associated with a rise in blood pressure, deterioration of renal function, anaemia, leuko-cytosis or a raised ESR (Akhtar *et al.*, 1972).

Pyelonephritis

This is the commonest renal disease in the elderly and affects men more than women. When chronic it is often asymptomatic or presents insidiously with the symptoms of uraemia: tiredness, anorexia, confusion, nausea and vomiting. In the acute episode there is loin pain, pyrexia, frequency and dysuria.

Treatment

Chronic bacteriuria is relatively benign, and although the urine may be temporarily sterilized by a course of antibiotics infection usually recurs and if asymptomatic is best ignored.

Acute infections should be treated along the usual lines, the choice of antibiotic depending upon the sensitivity of the organism. If symptoms are severe and treatment needs to be started before the result of culture is available then co-trimoxazole (Bactrim, Septrin) two tablets twice daily should be given. There is nothing to be gained by courses of antibiotics lasting longer than a week in uncomplicated urinary infections and, indeed, it has been shown in general practice that results of 10-day and 3-day treatments with amoxycillin 500 mg three times daily are the same.

In the presence of poor renal function the safest and most useful drugs are the penicillins, co-trimoxazole and gentamicin, because adequate urinary concentrations can be achieved without systemic toxicity (Asscher, 1977). Tetracyclines (except doxycycline, which is safe in normal doses: 100 mg once daily) must be avoided because their rapid accumulation leads to vomiting, diarrhoea and salt depletion which aggravates renal failure. They also have an anti-anabolic effect causing the blood urea to rise.

Nitrofurantoin is ineffective in renal failure and can cause irreversible peripheral neuropathy.

URINARY INCONTINENCE

The reported prevalence of incontinence varies considerably with the population surveyed and the criteria employed. A recent postal survey found that the prevalence of incontinence occurring twice or more a month was 7.6% for men and 12.5% for women aged 65 and over (Thomas *et al.*, 1978). In long-stay hospital patients the figure may be as high as 43% (Isaacs and Walkey, 1964) and here incontinence is not related to age, sex or duration of stay but to the presence of brain damage and whether the patient is able to dress, feed and walk independently.

Physiology of micturition

Despite a large literature on the subject there is still uncertainty about aspects of muscular control, innervation and even the anatomy of the bladder. Briefly, the bladder is under two nervous controls, the local reflex arc through the parasympathetic pelvic nerve (S2, 3 and 4) and voluntary control involving higher centres in the frontal cortex. As the bladder fills, sensory impulses pass along the afferent arc of the simple reflex and eventually the efferent arc to the detrusor is stimulated: there is coordinated contraction of the bladder and relaxation of periurethral striated muscle. Normally there is conscious awareness of bladder filling and the higher centre is able to inhibit local reflex contractions until time and place are appropriate for voluntary micturition (Brocklehurst, 1978).

With increasing age the higher centre control weakens so that, instead of being able to postpone micturition for an hour or more after the sensation of fulness has been experienced, an older person may only be able to delay micturition for a matter of minutes. If body and mind are sound the 'weak bladder' is catered for by certain precautions, such as restricting fluids before a long journey and micturating at frequent intervals. It is when mental function deteriorates or mobility declines that the trouble starts.

Causes of established incontinence

Neuropathic (neurogenic) bladders

Autonomous With destruction of the second to fourth sacral segments of the cauda equina (e.g. tumours, prolapsed discs or injury) there is loss of bladder sensation and emptying occurs from time to time due to intrinsic contractions. The anal–bulbocavernous reflex is absent and there may be painless bladder distension leading to overflow incontinence. The patient voids by straining and with the help of manual compression.

Atonic Lesions of the posterior nerve roots or posterior horn cells (as can occur in diabetes, tabes dorsalis, disseminated sclerosis, syringomyelia or sub-acute combined degeneration of the cord) produce a loss of bladder sensation and chronic distension: the result is retention with overflow.

Reflex A lesion between the sacral segments of the cord and higher centres (e.g. spinal injury, spinal cord tumours) will also cause loss of bladder sensation but the anal–bulbocavernous reflex is present. The bladder is unstable and empties reflexly, but the coordination is

217

lost and the external sphincter may fail to relax, producing high intravesical pressures.

Uninhibited   When there is damage to the higher centre or its connections in the cortex (e.g. dementia, strokes, fronto-parietal tumours) there is retention of sensation but the ability to inhibit reflex contractions is lost and the bladder becomes unstable. There may be urge incontinence where the patient's awareness of a desire to micturate is almost immediately followed by the passage of urine. However, the patient may retain continence and experience only urgency and nocturia.

Unstable bladder

This is a bladder which shows uninhibited contractions occurring at any capacity. These may happen during normal filling or following a rise in intra-abdominal pressure such as with coughing, laughing or standing up. This is a characteristic of reflex and uninhibited neuropathic bladders.

In both sexes there may be a congenital tendency toward an unstable bladder and such patients often have a childhood history of bed-wetting. In men, outflow obstruction due to an enlarged prostate or stricture may cause instability. Persistence of incontinence and urgency after prostatectomy is usually due to unrecognized instability.

Symptoms of an unstable bladder include frequency, nocturia, urgency, urge incontinence, stress incontinence and nocturnal enuresis.

Genuine stress incontinence

This is due to a mechanical or anatomical weakness of the urethral closure mechanism. It usually occurs during coughing or straining but the absence of other symptoms helps distinguish it from an unstable bladder. Only about half the patients with genuine stress incontinence actually leak when given the order to cough. It is most common in multiparous women and those with uterine prolapse, where it is often associated with deficiency in the striated muscle component of the pelvic floor. It is rare for the elderly to acquire

218

sphincter muscle weakness for the first time in old age. The initiating factor is thought to be hormonal changes accompanying childbirth.

Infection

Acute urinary infections may result in incontinence but it is a fairly unusual cause. Chronic urinary infection does not lead to incontinence.

Urethritis

The urethra is derived from the mesodermal Woolfian system and contains oestrogen-sensitive epithelium. Oestrogen deficiency not only produces atrophic vaginitis, recognized clinically as a reddened sore vagina, with a red, speckled cervix, but causes a urethritis with dysuria and incontinence.

Transient incontinence

Anything that disorientates, confuses or renders the patient bedfast is likely to cause incontinence. Thus it is a common accompaniment to most acute illnesses in the elderly, particularly if they suddenly find themselves in the strange surroundings of a hospital.

Drugs

Diuretics given to a poorly mobile patient are very likely to produce incontinence. Heavily sedated patients will not be able to wake up and use the lavatory and anticholinergic drugs (including the tricyclic antidepressants) may cause retention with overflow.

Investigating incontinence

Patients should be divided into those with transient and those with established incontinence. There should be a full history and review of drugs followed by physical examination, including a rectal and

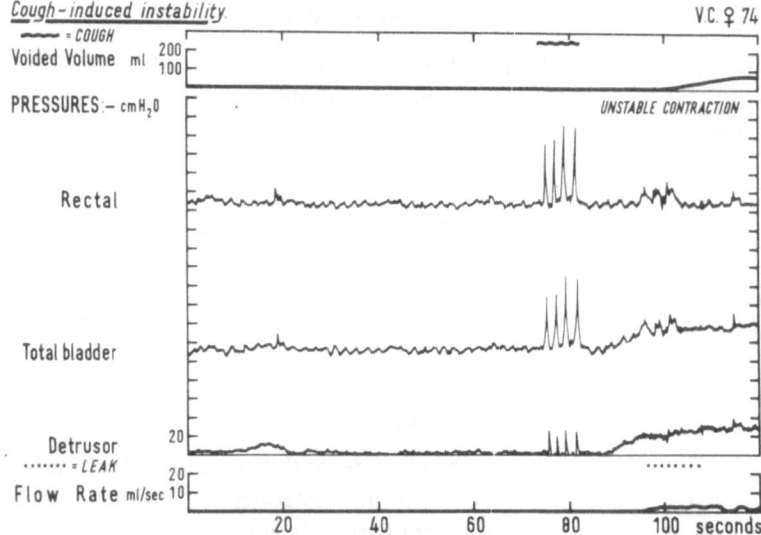

Figure 1 Cough-induced instability. Following a cough there is an unstable bladder contraction with leakage of urine. This is *not* genuine stress incontinence.

vaginal examination. Urine culture (MSU) is the minimum investigation but ideally all patients, with the exception of those severely handicapped by strokes or dementia, should have a voiding cystometrogram (VCMG)* (Figures 1–4).

VCMG gives a true recording of the intravesical pressure and allows measurement of total bladder capacity, volume at which the desire to void occurs, response to stress (such as coughing), voiding, pressure and flow rates. Video-cysto-urethrography may be combined with VCMG to give a simultaneous picture of the bladder. If this is unavailable a simple micturating cystogram can give useful information (see Table 1).

Voiding cystometrograms. A thin catheter connected to a pressure sensitive transducer is passed into the rectum and another into the bladder. Rectal pressure corresponds to the pressure in the abdomen and is automatically subtracted from the total bladder pressure to give 'pure' detrusor pressure. The rate at which urine is passed is shown by the flow rate and the total amount measured as the voided volume.

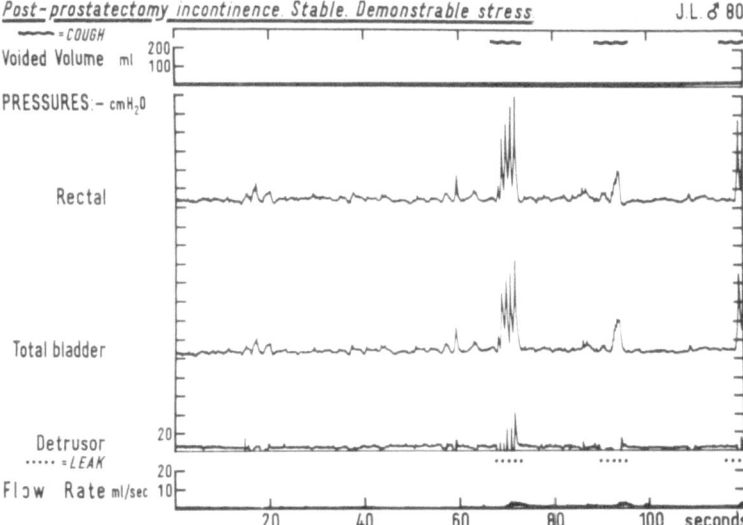

Figure 2 Post-prostatectomy incontinence. The bladder is stable, but there is stress incontinence shown by leakage of urine coinciding with the cough.

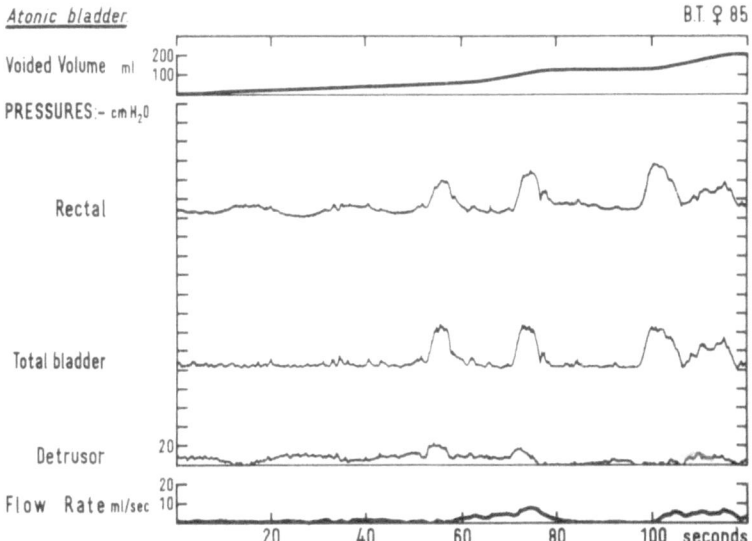

Figure 3 Atonic bladder. The patient, who has diabetes mellitus, is straining to pass urine, shown by rises in abdominal (rectal) and total bladder pressure but the detrusor contractions are poor and little urine is passed.

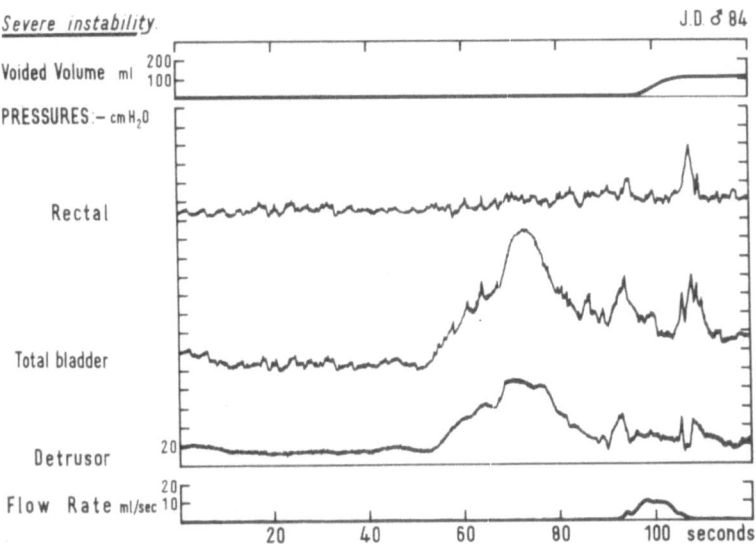

Figure 4 Severe instability. The patient is demented and unstable bladder contractions are occurring spontaneously during bladder filling resulting in incontinence.

TABLE 1
RADIOLOGICAL APPEARANCE OF THE BLADDER

	Neuropathic	*Unstable*
Shape	Fir tree	Normal
Trabeculation	+++	±
Residual urine	++	±

Where atrophic vaginitis is suspected a vaginal smear should be taken to assess the maturation of cells in the vaginal wall: this is related to the amount of oestrogen present.

Not only does proper investigation of incontinence provide a diagnosis but it allows all staff concerned (and the patient himself) to see that incontinence is not a mysterious, inevitable accompaniment of ageing but a problem with clearly defined causes.

222

Treatment

Transient incontinence nearly always disappears as the patient's general condition improves and as he familiarizes himself with his new surroundings. Avoidance of drugs likely to aggravate incontinence and an emphasis on improving mobility are important.

Bladder training

In many patients with an unstable bladder, from whatever cause, incontinence can be minimized by retraining. The nurse records on a chart (4- or 2-hourly) whether the patient is wet or dry and helps him to use the lavatory or commode. After a day or two the patient's pattern of incontinence can be recognized and the nurse then tries to forstall incontinence by getting the patient to pass urine before he has wet himself. The mere act of filling in a chart and the consequent interest in the patient's bladder function encourages self-respect, and once he is dry (albeit with frequent assisted visits to the lavatory) there is often a considerable improvement in morale and well-being. The importance of regular toileting must be explained to the relatives as well as the patient, since the new habit will have to be maintained at home.

Drugs

The most widely used at present are the anticholinergic type, although they are far from satisfactory. The rationale is that unstable bladder contractions are parasympathetic in origin and may be suppressed by anticholinergic activity. Such drugs should not be used where there is glaucoma or prostatic obstruction. Emepromium bromide (Ceteprin) is given in a dose of 400 mg at night and up to 200 mg three times daily by day.

Propantheline and flavoxate hydrochloride (Urispas) have a direct relaxant effect on the bladder and are probably equally effective.

Prostaglandins E and F cause bladder contraction and may have a physiological function. Prostaglandin antagonists (e.g. Indomethecin) have been used successfully and are being further investigated.

223

Another approach is to look at the effect of calcium antagonists (e.g. verapamil, nifedipine) in preventing uptake of calcium by the contracting detrusor.

Genuine stress incontinence
Here it is vital to get the diagnosis right and to exclude those with abnormal bladder function. When the diagnosis is established the first step is to persuade the obese to lose weight. The wearing of corsets should be stopped and chronic cough treated where possible. Oestrogens have a direct effect on the mucosal lining of the urinary tract and possibly on smooth muscle as well.

Ethinyl oestradiol 10 μg or dienoestrol cream are often helpful in tending to reduce frequency, nocturia and incontinence.

Physiotherapy exercises to strengthen the pubo-coccygeus are also effective. The method is explained to the patient and she is warned that beneficial effects may take some time to appear and that the exercises are tiring. She is instructed to relax and to control her pelvic floor muscles in a controlled, steady manner. She must practise stopping and starting the flow in mid-stream.

Finally, surgery may need to be considered. The aim is to provide a firm shelf under the urethra against which the occlusive force that closes the urethra can act. Surgery is not much help in the elderly unless there is a gross prolapse.

Urethritis and atrophic vaginitis
Oestrogens are the specific treatment. The oral form is best since dienoestrol cream may be difficult for the elderly patient to use and results in the same blood levels. Ethinyl oestradiol 10 μg should be given in three-weekly courses. There is a risk of endometrial bleeding.

Atonic bladder
Cholinergic drugs are often useful. Bethanacol chloride can be given subcutaneously (not i.v. or i.m.), initially in a dose of 2.5–5.0 mg repeated three or four times daily and then an oral dose of 10–15 mg three times daily is substituted. Distigmine bromide (Ubretid) can be used instead in oral doses of 5 mg daily or 0.5 ml i.m. If drugs are inef-

fective the patient should be taught to empty his bladder by a combination of straining and manual compression.

Catheters

Although not the first-line treatment of incontinence, catheters should not be regarded as the ultimate horror. Many patients, dry for the first time in years, are very pleased with their indwelling catheter. The patient should be taught how to empty and change the drainage bag and should be given a 'Shepheard's sporran' (Medical Supply Association Ltd.) or similar device whereby the bag is out of sight and suspended comfortably from the waist.

Chronic urinary infection is common but is not usually a problem to the elderly patient with a long-term indwelling catheter. Neither continuous urinary antiseptics nor short courses of antibiotics are helpful. Weekly bladder washouts with 1% noxyflex may reduce the amount of catheter blockage and the resultant leakage. Despite the claims made for silastic catheters there is little difference in practice between the times *in situ* for silastic and latex Foley catheters (Brocklehurst and Brocklehurst 1978).

Appliances

There is a wide range of incontinence pads and pants, sheaths for males and specially designed clothes for both sexes. These are well described by Mandelstam (1977) and can be seen at the Disabled Living Foundation, Kensington High Street, London. It is essential that anyone regularly seeing incontinent patients should know what appliances are available and be able to select the most suitable one for the individual. Proper fitting is important, and this should ideally be done by a specially trained nurse working closely with an Incontinence Clinic, who is available to give advice to patients, relatives, residential home staff and community nurses.

BENIGN PROSTATIC HYPERTROPHY

With age, small areas in the prostate gland grow and coalesce into adenomata. The process is irreversible and probably triggered by hormonal changes. Outflow obstruction leads to trabeculation and thickening of the bladder wall, the ureters dilate and vesico-ureteric reflux occurs. The size of the prostate, however, is not related to the degree of outflow destruction.

Clinical features

These include frequency, poor stream, hesitancy and acute or chronic retention. There may be a remarkable absence of symptoms and sometimes the only indication of retention with overflow is nocturnal enuresis; 40% of men with obstructive outflow symptoms have an unstable bladder but most do well with prostatectomy. Incontinence is rare following operation, and if it does occur is usually due to persisting bladder instability.

The differential diagnosis of prostatism includes carcinoma of the prostate or bladder (frequency mimicking outflow obstruction without haematuria may be the presenting symptom), depression, the sideeffects of anticholinergic drugs, a prolapsed disc causing a highpressure bladder with retention of urine and polyuria due to atrophy of the renal parenchyma (characterized by the passage of large quantities of isotonic urine at night).

Investigations will include culture of urine, measurement of blood sugar, urea, creatinine and electrolytes and an intravenous pyelogram.

Treatment

Generally speaking it is better to operate early rather than late, and advanced age should not be a deterrent. The development of uraemia is often insidious causing gradually increasing confusion and apathy. Infection of residual urine, uraemia, and a floppy atonic bladder not only increase the operative mortality but also lessen the chances of a good result. Patients who develop acute or chronic retention are also a poor operative risk. They may be salt and water depleted, acidotic, or anaemic. Correction of dehydration and transfusion prior to prostatectomy is essential (Blandy, 1974).

226

CARCINOMA OF THE PROSTATE

Over the age of 90 nearly all prostates contain a focus of carcinoma.

Included in the assessment should be an assay of the prostatic acid phosphatase (only 25% of cases with tumour confined to the prostate have raised levels, compared with 75% where there are metastases or extracapsular spread), alkaline phosphatase, chest X-ray and bone scan.

A transurethral resection may be needed for obstructive symptoms and possibly hormone treatment or radiotherapy. Oestrogens are effective in relieving pain due to bony metastases and reducing serum acid phosphatase levels. Small doses (stilboestrol 1 mg three times daily) produce the same improvement as a larger dose and have less side-effects.

HYPONATRAEMIA

This is commonly found in elderly people admitted to hospital but is rarely diagnosed clinically. The symptoms are non-specific and include mental confusion, lassitude, anorexia, nausea and headache. It is likely that hyponatraemia is responsible for the majority of such symptoms in patients whose serum sodium is less than 125 mmol/l (mEq/l).

The causes of hyponatraemia can be divided into:

(1) Primary salt depletion (e.g. sweating, diarrhoea, diuretics, and adrenocortical insufficiency).
(2) Water intoxication (e.g. congestive cardiac failure, cirrhosis, renal failure and SIADH (see Chapter 11).

One recent report on severe hyponatraemia that excluded patients with severe heart failure, acute renal failure or endocrine deficiency, found an iatrogenic cause in 41% of cases. They were mainly due to prolonged diuretic therapy, use of 5% dextrose i.v. following surgery or both. Bacterial chest infections were more commonly to blame than carcinoma of the bronchus. Analyses of blood and urine were of no value in distinguishing the diagnostic groups in an emergency. The hyponatraemia and relevant symptoms cleared rapidly when diuretics or i.v. dextrose were stopped, chest infections treated or salt and water losses replaced (Kennedy, Mitchell and Hoffbrand, 1978).

Thiazides, loop diuretics and Moduretic (hydrochlorothiazide 50 mg and amiloride 5 mg) have all been reported to cause hyponatraemia. It appears that the elderly are particularly at risk and that the intensity of treatment is more relevant than the type of diuretic.

ACUTE RENAL FAILURE

The elderly make up only a small percentage of the referrals to renal units, yet it has been found that the prognosis is not dependent on age alone: the mortality in acute renal failure is between 50 and 60% irrespective of age.

The major factor in the development of acute renal failure is dehydration and electrolyte imbalance (Kumar, Hill and McGeown, 1973). The elderly patient with impaired renal function is particularly at risk from inadequate fluid intake and hyponatraemia and hypokalaemia due to diuretics. Profound hypotension following major surgery, myocardial infarction or gastrointestinal haemorrhage is another important cause, as is toxaemia secondary to bronchopneumonia and the incautious use of tetracyclines.

In most cases a successful outcome follows correction of fluid and electrolyte imbalance, with routine care of the bladder, prevention of superinfection and dietary control. Antibiotics are best reserved for proven infections and used under bacteriological control. In only about a quarter of cases is dialysis needed. Deaths are usually the result of infection, particularly bronchopneumonia, or myocardial infarction.

REFERENCES

Akhtar, A. J., Andrews, G. R., Caird, F. I. and Fallon R. J. (1972). Urinary tract infection in the elderly: a population study. *Age and Ageing*, **1**, 48

Urogenital system

Asscher, A. W. (1977). Diseases of the urinary system: urinary tract infections. *Br. Med. J.*, **1,** 1332

Blandy, J. (1974). Management of benign enlargement of the prostate, *Br. J. Hosp. Med.*, **11,** 375

Brocklehurst, J. C. (1978). The investigation and management of incontinence. In B. Isaacs (ed.). *Recent Advances in Geriatric Medicine*. (Edinburgh: Churchill Livingstone)

Brocklehurst, J. C., Dillane, J. B., Griffiths, L. L. and Fry, J. (1968). The prevalence and symptomatology of urinary infection in an aged population, *Geront. Clin.*, **10,** 242

Brocklehurst, J. C., Fry, J., Griffiths, L. L. and Kalton, G. (1972). Urinary infection and symptoms of dysuria in women aged 45–64 years: their relevance to similar findings in the elderly. *Age and Ageing*, **1,** 41

Brocklehurst, J. C. and Brocklehurst, S. (1978). The management of indwelling catheters. *Br. J. Urol.*, **50,** 102

Denham, M. J., Hodkinson, H. M. and Fisher, M. (1975). Glomerular filtration rate in sick elderly inpatients. *Age and Ageing*, **4,** 32

Hodkinson, H. M. (1978). The interpretation of biochemical data. In B. Isaacs (ed.). *Recent Advances in Geriatric Medicine*. (Edinburgh: Churchill Livingstone)

Isaacs, B. and Walkey, F. A. (1964). A survey of incontinence in elderly hospital patients, *Geront. Clin.*, **6,** 367

Kennedy, P. G. E., Mitchell, D. M. and Hoffbrand, B. I. (1978). Severe hyponatraemia in hospital in-patients. *Br. Med. J.*, **2,** 1251

Kumar, R., Hill, C. M. and McGeown, M. G. (1973). Acute renal failure in the elderly. *Lancet*, **i,** 90

Lapides, J. and Costello, R. T. (1969). Uninhibited neurogenic bladder: a common cause for recurrent urinary tract infection in normal women. *J. Urol.*, **101,** 539

Mandelstam, D. (1977). *Incontinence*. (London: Disabled Living Foundation)

McLachlan, M. S. F. (1978). The ageing kidney. *Lancet*, **ii,** 143

Thomas, T. M., Plymat, K. R., Blannin, J. and Meade, T. W. (1978). *The Prevalence of Incontinence in the Community*. VIIIth International Continence Society Meeting. (Oxford: Pergamon Press)

11
Endocrine disorders

Studies on the ageing of endocrine glands are few and tend to be contradictory, reflecting the difficulty in distinguishing between physiological changes and the effect of diseases.

In the thyroid the follicles are smaller with a corresponding reduction in colloid and increase in volume of epithelial cells. Fibrous connective tissue between the follicles is increased. Although thyroid function declines with age there is no correlation between function and histological changes.

In the pancreas little alteration has been noted in the secretory cells with age other than an increased variation in their appearance and an accumulation of pigment. Physiological changes in thyroid function and glucose metabolism are described later.

THYROID DISEASE

Although thyroxine (T_4) is the main hormone produced by the thyroid gland and present in the serum it is much less metabolically active than triiodothyronine (T_3). T_3 is formed by conversion from T_4 and

231

the serum levels are very much lower than those of T_4.

Ageing is associated with a decline in T_3 of about 5.1 ng/100 ml every 10 years (Rubenstein, Butler and Werner, 1973). This is probably not due to a decrease in thyroid-binding globulin (TBG) and may represent a change in output of T_3 by the thyroid, a reduced peripheral conversion of T_4 to T_3 or an increased rate of utilization. In this study no change was found in serum T_4 levels and Hodkinson and Denham (1977) have confirmed this finding in healthy elderly subjects. However Britton *et al.* (1975) concluded that serum T_4 did rise with age and that 'T_4 toxicosis' in elderly female hospital patients is primarily a biochemical finding.

One of the difficulties in interpreting thyroid function tests in the elderly is that very often the patient is ill, with a corresponding fall in both serum albumin and TBG, probably due to impaired liver synthesis (Jefferys *et al.*, 1972). This means that an isolated estimation of serum T_4 may be unreliable and the free thyroxine index (FTI) is widely used as a means of improving accuracy. The FTI gives an indirect assessment of free thyroxine and is calculated by dividing serum T_4 by T_3 uptake and multiplying by a hundred. Sick elderly inpatients have a much wider range FTI (0.54–1.59) than well elderly subjects living at home (0.58–1.24) (Hodkinson and Denham, 1977).

The importance of illness in distorting laboratory tests of thyroid function is further emphasized by Burrows *et al.* (1975). They examined 79 euthyroid elderly patients and found that 59% of inpatients and 10% of outpatients had low serum T_3 levels. In contrast 12% and 30% respectively had a raised serum T_4. TSH levels were significantly lower than in young adult controls. Further investigation of the fall in serum T_3 during illness was carried out by Chopra *et al.* (1975) who showed that as serum T_3 fell, levels of reverse T_3 (rT_3) increased. This suggests that the peripheral conversion of T_4 to rT_3 and T_3 represents two distinct competitive routes. Whether this is a defence reaction of the body under stress to generate poorly calorigenic rT_3 instead of the very potent T_3, or is an abnormality of T_4 metabolism that simply reflects generalized illness, is not yet clear. The change is reversible. Modest elevations of the FTI, due to a raised serum T_4, occur in many apparently euthyroid elderly patients and may be caused by drugs such as L-dopa, digoxin and co-trimoxazole (Baruch, Davis and Hodkinson, 1976).

Prevalence

It will be seen from the foregoing discussion that estimates of prevalence of thyroid disease in an elderly population depend upon the criteria adopted for determining the normal range of thyroid function tests. Generally it is accepted that the prevalence of unsuspected thyroid disease, mainly hypothyroidism, is 2–3%, both in hospital patients and well elderly subjects in the community. This probably justifies routine screening in ill old people. However, routine screening of 662 admissions to a psychogeriatric unit over a 6-year period found hypothyroidism in 1.2% and hyperthyroidism in 0.76%.In only two patients was thyroid disease considered to be a significant factor in the psychiatric presentation and it was felt that the practical benefits resulting from screening were so disappointing as to not justify it (Henschke and Pain, 1977).

Hypothyroidism

Clinical features

It appears that less than one-third of previously unsuspected cases have the classical signs and symptoms of hypothyroidism. Far more commonly there is a non-specific picture of declining mobility and general health. In about a quarter of patients there is a relevant associated disease (such as rheumatoid arthritis or pernicious anaemia) and in another quarter a psychosis other than dementia, usually depression or paranoia (Bahemuka and Hodkinson, 1975). Psychiatric symptoms have been a well-recognized feature of hypothyroidism since Asher (1949) described 'myxoedematous madness'. His 14 cases had a non-specific psychosis where paranoid ideas were common. Such a florid presentation is fairly rare though, and it is more usual to find impairment of cognitive function and/or depression. Other features include a liability to develop hypothermia (see Chapter 5), deafness, polyarthralgia, macrocytosis and falls.

233

Diagnosis

The FTI is a useful screening test although TSH assay has greater discriminatory power and should be used for confirmation. In primary hypothyroidism TSH levels are high, although raised levels are also seen in euthyroid patients who have had radioactive iodine treatment or thyroidectomy. Inappropriately low levels with a persistently low FTI indicate secondary hypothyroidism. This should be investigated with the thyrotropin-releasing hormone (TRH) test, where 400 µg of TRH are injected intravenously and serum TSH levels measured over the next 2 hours. Failure of serum TSH levels to rise is seen in pituitary disease, whereas a normal increase in serum TSH indicates a hypothalamic disorder. Care is needed in interpreting the response since it has been shown that in men (but not in women) there is a marked fall in TSH response with increasing age (Snyder and Utiger, 1972a and b).

Treatment

Thyroxine 0.05 mg daily is the starting dose and is gradually increased according to the patient's response and falling serum TSH level. In patients with ischaemic heart disease the dose should be raised very cautiously, not more frequently than every fortnight. Mild impairment of cognitive function (but not established dementia), apathy, 'failure to thrive', deafness and macrocytosis can all be expected to improve with treatment. For patients with hypothermia due to hypothyroidism, tri-iodothyronine 20 µg 4-hourly has been recommended, but its value is doubtful.

Hyperthyroidism

Clinical features

Again, atypical presentation is usual. Thyrotoxic symptoms are less pronounced in the elderly and features such as hot, sweaty hands, hyperkinesis and thyroid gland bruit are frequently absent. Instead, heart failure and uncontrolled atrial fibrillation are common, as are apathy, confusion and depression. Elderly women are particularly susceptible to osteoporosis secondary to thyrotoxicosis and have an increased incidence of fractures.

Diagnosis

A high serum T_4 and FTI is nearly always found, but false positive results due to drugs such as L-dopa can occur (*vide supra*). Doubtful results can be confirmed by measuring the serum T_3 or radioactive technetium uptake.

Treatment

Radioactive iodine is usually the treatment of first choice in the elderly. Its main drawback is subsequent hypothyroidism, which occurs in up to 35% of patients. Alternatively carbimazole 10 mg three times daily may be given with the addition of a beta-blocker if necessary. After 6 months the drug should be discontinued to see if toxicity has abated.

DIABETES MELLITUS

With increasing age glomerular filtration rate falls and renal glucose threshold rises. Thus many patients with hyperglycaemia will not have glycosuria. However, those that do (especially women) are very likely to have an abnormal glucose tolerance test (GTT) (Butterfield, 1964). Glucose tolerance is impaired with age and it is difficult to know if this is physiological and whether one should therefore alter one's criteria for the diagnosis of diabetes. It is probably best, regardless of age, to regard a 2-hour blood sugar above 6.7 mmol/l (120 mg/100 ml) as abnormal, although whether it should be treated is another matter. In practice a random blood sugar is the most convenient way of screening new patients and a level above 10.4 mmol/l (187 mg/100 ml) will include the majority of diabetics and very few non-diabetics (Denham, 1972).

Clinical features

As in younger age groups there may be thirst, polyuria and pruritus. Presentation with complications or with incontinence related to polyuria and immobility is common in the elderly. Frequently the diagnosis is only made as a result of routine screening. Gangrene due to peripheral vascular disease may be seen, and also deep painless ulcers if there is a peripheral neuropathy. The neuropathy is usually symmetrical and in addition to the loss of vibration sense and lower limb reflexes, which is common in old age, there is also loss of pain and light touch sensation. Amyotrophy can cause pain, weakness and wasting of hip and thigh muscles. It may be so severe that the patient is unable to rise from a chair, but the prospects for recovery are fairly good if the diabetes is controlled. Vision is often impaired by retinopathy or cataracts.

Confusion, irrational behaviour or coma in a diabetic patient raises the possibility of hypoglycaemia and this is particularly likely in patients on long-acting hypoglycaemic drugs who forget meals. Hyperglycaemic coma often follows a precipitating illness, such as an infection, but may occur for the first time in a mild diabetic for no apparent reason. In elderly patients coma is usually preceded by a relatively asymptomatic stage: thirst, tiredness, failure to cope and then a sudden loss of consciousness.

Hyperosmolar non-hepatic coma occurs most frequently in the elderly. There is usually no obvious cause, but diuretics, steroids, pancreatitis or extensive burns may precipitate coma. There is no smell of acetone on the patient's breath and polyuria and thirst are prominent. The blood sugar is raised and bicarbonate is in the normal range or just below.

Treatment

Most patients who are relatively free from symptoms and have a blood sugar of less than 16–17 mmol/l (300 mg/100 ml) can be controlled on diet alone. It is often difficult to persuade the patient to keep to a diet and any regime must be simple. For the obese, non-insulin-dependent diabetic the aim is simply to restrict calories and for the non-obese patient to restrict carbohydrate. If the intention is to restrict carbohydrate to 40% of the diet then the number of grams required represents one-tenth of the total calorie intake. Thus on a

1200 calorie diet, 12 g of carbohydrate would be the maximum permitted. However, some elderly people eat mostly carbohydrate because it is cheap, and the carbohydrate content can then be increased to 60% of the diet with a consequent reduction in fat.

If a hypoglycaemic drug is needed the most useful and the safest is tolbutamide 500 mg–2 g daily in divided doses. The long-acting chlorpropamide is best avoided because of the risk of hypoglycaemia. If a sulphonylurea fails to give adequate control then a biguanide should be added and metformin 0.5–1.5 g daily is the drug of choice. The risk of lactic acidosis with phenformin makes its use unjustified in most circumstances. Insulin is best given as a single morning dose using one of the long-acting preparations such as isophane (NPH). This starts to act after about an hour, reaches a peak between 8 and 12 hours and tails off by 24 hours. A small dose (e.g. 16 units) may be used initially and the amount gradually increased, ensuring that the early evening blood sugar (when the insulin is exerting its maximum effect) does not fall below 8.3 mmol/l (150 mg/100 ml). The aim is to achieve reasonable control without producing hypoglycaemia and quite high blood sugars of around 15 mmol/l (270 mg/100 ml) may be tolerated. During intercurrent illness, when control is often lost, it is best to switch to twice- or thrice-daily injections of soluble insulin, trying to avoid hypoglycaemia and the reactive peaks of hyperglycaemia.

Hyperglycaemia coma is managed in the same way as in younger patients. In addition to i.v. infusions of N saline and potassium, soluble insulin is given in an initial i.m. dose of 10–20 units and then 5 units i.m. hourly until the blood sugar is in the region of 8–18 mmol/l (144–324 mg/100 ml). Alternatively soluble insulin may be given in small doses (3–6 units/hour) by continuous i.v. infusion. It is probably best to give a broad-spectrum antibiotic to all patients in hyperglycaemic coma.

Hyperosmolar non-ketotic acidosis produces a severe dehydration and patients need, in addition to small doses of insulin, large amounts of hypotonic glucose/saline (5–10 l in the first 24 hours).

Also of importance in the management of the diabetic is early referral to an ophthalmic or vascular surgeon if poor visual acuity is present or gangrene threatens. The patient should be taught how to care for his skin and feet, with help from the community nurse or chiropodist if necessary.

SYNDROME OF INAPPROPRIATE ANTIDIURETIC HORMONE (SIADH)

This is only one cause of hyponatraemia (see Chapter 10) and must be distinguished from excessive use of diuretics, congestive cardiac failure, cirrhosis of the liver and secondary adrenocortical insufficiency. It is characterized by a low serum osmolality and, simultaneously, urine less than maximally dilute. The hyponatraemia persists even when large quantities of sodium are given and is corrected by vigorous water restriction alone (de Troyer and Demanet, 1976). Clinically these patients are distinguished from those with salt depletion (e.g. Addison's disease) by being relatively fit (despite the hyponatraemia), well-hydrated, normotensive, with a normal haematocrit and a normal or low blood urea.

The syndrome may be seen with cerebral tumours, strokes, carcinoma of the bronchus, bronchopneumonia, hypothyroidism, tumours of the gastrointestinal tract and drugs such as chlorpropamide, clofibrate, barbiturates, morphine and diuretics. The syndrome does not respond to sodium replacement and severe restriction of water is needed. As a temporary measure in acute cases this is acceptable, but where the condition is prolonged, frusemide, which can produce a dilute urine in hyponatraemic oedematous patients, is given together with a small volume of hypotonic (3%) saline to replace urinary electrolytes loss (*N. Engl. J. Med.*, Leader, 1978).

REFERENCES

Asher, R. (1949). Myxoedematous madness. *Br. Med. J.*, **2**, 555
Bahemuka, M. and Hodkinson, H. M. (1975). Screening for hypothyroidism in elderly patients. *Br. Med. J.*, **2**, 601
Baruch, A. L. H., Davis, C. and Hodkinson, H. M. (1976). Causes of high

free-thyroxine-index values in sick euthyroid elderly patients. *Age and Ageing*, **5**, 224

Britton, K. E., Quinn, V., Ellis, S. M., Cayley, A. C. D., Miralles, J. M., Brown, B. L. and Ekins, R. P. (1975). Is 'T-toxicosis' a normal biochemical finding in elderly women? *Lancet*, **ii**, 141

Burrows, A. W., Shakespear, R. A., Hesch, R. D., Cooper, E., Aickin, C. M. and Burke, C. W. (1975). Thyroid hormones in the elderly sick: 'T$_4$-euthyroidism'. *Br. Med. J.*, **4**, 437

Butterfield, W. J. H. (1964). Summary of results of the Bedford diabetes survey. *Proc. Roy. Soc. Med*, **57**, 196

Chopra, I. J., Chopra, U., Smith, S. R., Reza, M. and Solomon, D. H. (1975). Reciprocal changes in serum concentrations of 3,3',5'-triiodothyronine (reverse T$_3$) and 3,3',5-triiodothyronine (T$_3$) in systemic illnesses. *Clin. Endocrinol. Metab.*, **41**, 1043

Denham, M. J. (1972). The value of random blood glucose determinations as a screening method for detecting diabetes mellitus in the elderly patient. *Age and Ageing*, **1**, 55

De Troyer, A., and Demanet, J. C. (1976). Clinical, biological and pathogenic features of the syndrome of inappropriate secretion of antidiuretic hormone. *Q. J. Med., N.S.*, **45**, 521

Henschke, P. J. and Pain, R. W. (1977). Thyroid disease in a psychogeriatric population. *Age and Ageing*, **6**, 151

Hodkinson, H. M. and Denham, M. J. (1977). Thyroid function tests in the elderly in the community. *Age and Ageing*, **6**, 67

Jefferys, P. M., Farran, H. E. A., Hoffenberg, R., Fraser, P. M. and Hodkinson, H. M. (1972). Thyroid function tests in the elderly. *Lancet*, **i**, 924

Leader (1978). New treatments for hyponatraemia. *N. Engl. J. Med.* **298**, 214

Rubenstein, H. A., Butler, V. P. and Werner, S. C. (1973). Progressive decrease in serum triiodothyronine concentration with human ageing: radio-immunoassay following extraction of serum. *J. Clin. Endocrinol. Metab.*, **37**, 247

Snyder, P. J. and Utiger, R. D. (1972a). Response to thyrotropin releasing hormone (TRH) in normal man. *J. Clin. Endocrinol. Metab.*, **34**, 380

Snyder, P. J. and Utiger, R. D. (1972b). Thyrotropin response to thyrotropin releasing hormone in normal females over forty. *J. Clin. Endocrinol. Metab.*, **34**, 1096

12

Blood disorders

AGEING

Ageing has remarkably little effect on blood constituents. The life span of erythrocytes is unaltered and there are only very minor changes in the leukocyte count. With increasing age albumen falls and globulins rise, which probably accounts, in part, for increased values of the erythrocyte sedimentation rate (ESR).

Erythrocyte sedimentation rate (ESR)

The red-cell sedimentation rate is often found to be raised in normal, healthy elderly people and is attributed to the fall in albumen and rise in globulins that occur with increasing age. Plasma viscosity is usually normal on these occasions. ESRs of up to 45 mm/h in both sexes are commonplace and although frequently no cause can be found, persistently high values should raise the possibility of polymyalgia rheumatica, giant cell arteritis or myeloma. The other causes of a raised ESR that can occur in younger patients must also be considered.

ANAEMIA

The normal range of haemoglobin is unaltered by age, so that a haemoglobin of less than 12.0 g/100 ml in an elderly person should not be

241

dismissed as being 'physiological'. Most surveys have shown that the prevalence of anaemia increases with age and is higher in women than in men. One random urban survey on people over the age of 65 (Parsons *et al.*, 1965) found that when anaemia was defined as less than 12.5 g/100 ml for men and 12.0 g/100 ml for women, 10.8% of men and 15.7% of women were anaemic. One consequence of taking an arbitary dividing line of haemoglobin values to define anaemia is that normal subjects can fall below this line. Among elderly anaemic patients McLennan *et al.* (1973) found no cause for the anaemia in 30%. Almost all were women and had a haemoglobin just below 12 g/100 ml.

Iron deficiency anaemia

This accounts for 45% of elderly anaemic patients (McLennan *et al.*, 1973). Blood loss from the gastrointestinal tract is usually responsible and may be due to hiatus hernia, peptic ulceration, diverticular disease, haemorrhoids, malignant disease or gastric erosions caused by drugs such as aspirin and indomethacin. In up to 16% of patients no cause for the bleeding may be found (Beveridge *et al.*, 1965). Many patients have no gastric symptoms, and several stool tests for occult blood may be needed before a positive result is found. The presence of a minor degree of malabsorption (usually coeliac disease) can cause iron deficiency anaemia and although obvious steatorrhoea is unusual, laboratory estimation of the faecal fat content, as well as evidence of other deficiencies, may be helpful in making a diagnosis. Partial gastrectomy will also result in malabsorption of iron. The incidence of achlorhydria increases with age (Beveridge *et al.*, 1965) and in most cases gastric parietal cell antibodies are present. When both antibodies and achlorhydria occur the risk of developing pernicious anaemia is 32%. Overall 6% of patients with iron deficiency anaemia have coexisting pernicious anaemia (Dagg *et al.*, 1966). The importance of malnutrition as a cause of iron deficiency anaemia in the elderly has probably been overemphasized, although the intake of both iron and calories does fall with age (Hallberg and Högdahl, 1971).

Nevertheless a full dietary history is worth taking. Miscellaneous causes include infections, chronic renal failure, rheumatoid arthritis and malignant disease.

Clinical features

Elderly patients often present with a non-specific decline in their general health. There may be a history of gradually increasing confusion, apathy, self-neglect, a failure to cope at home and frequent falls. Dyspnoea, dizziness and tiredness may be present and heart failure frequently accompanies severe anaemia. The mucous membranes are always pale, although a blepharitis may mislead if only the lower eyelid is examined. Atrophic glossitis is a more reliable sign than angular stomatitis, but both conditions are quite common in normal elderly people.

Investigations

The Coulter 'S' counter gives an accurate measure of haemoglobin and blood indices, but estimates of iron reserves from the serum iron and total iron binding capacity are unreliable in ill patients. The serum iron can fall very rapidly following an acute infection and both measurements can be depressed in the presence of carcinomatosis and chronic renal failure. In addition serum iron falls with age. The most accurate way to assess total iron stores is to measure the serum ferritin or the stainable iron on a marrow smear. A thorough search for the cause of the iron deficiency should be made, and will include tests for blood in faeces and urine, blood urea and creatinine, faecal fat, sigmoidoscopy, chest X-ray, barium studies and an intravenous pyelogram.

Treatment

Many patients relapse after treatment, and the difficulties of treating iron deficiency in the elderly are similar to those in younger patients (see Table 1). Oral therapy with ferrous sulphate (400–600 mg a day in divided doses) will, depending on the degree of anaemia, return the haemoglobin to normal in 6–8 weeks. However, treatment should continue for another 3 months to replenish iron stores. Common side-effects include nausea, diarrhoea, constipation and epigastric pain but there is no difference in their frequency between ferrous sulphate, fumarate or carbonate. If the patient complains of symptoms he should be advised to take the tablets after meals and halve the dose for a while. Changing the iron preparation to a tablet with a different colour or to one of the slow-release capsule is occasionally effective.

TABLE 1

CAUSES OF TREATMENT FAILURE IN IRON DEFICIENCY ANAEMIA

1. Inadequate treatment of underlying condition e.g. blood loss continues

2. Non-compliance
   (a) Doctor failed to give adequate instructions
   (b) Troublesome side-effects
   (c) Patient's confusion or lack of interest

3. Anaemia due to other causes
   e.g. B_{12} or folate deficiency, sideroblastic anaemia, myeloma

A patient who cannot be relied upon to take his tablets should be considered for parenteral iron. Use of the intramuscular or intravenous route does not produce a faster rise in haemoglobin, but it does ensure that the iron gets into the patient. Iron sorbitol citrate (Jectofer) is given intramuscularly in a dose of 2 ml (100 mg of iron), which raises the haemoglobin by about 0.4 g/100 ml. The dose is usually repeated on alternate days until the total necessary to raise the haemoglobin to normal levels, plus 1 g for the stores, has been given. Apart from local irritation, allergic reactions and a metallic taste in the mouth the main practical difficulty is buttocks that are insufficiently fleshy to take the repeated injections.

Now well established is the use of iron dextran by total dose infusion. This must not be given to patients with asthma or a history of allergy since severe hypersensitivity reactions can be provoked. The total dose of iron is calculated and added to 500 ml of 5% dextrose. The intravenous infusion is run in no faster than 10 drops a minute for 10 minutes with adrenaline and resuscitation equipment immediately available. If no reaction occurs the infusion can be speeded up. The commonest side-effect in one series of elderly patients was local phlebitis (Wright, 1967) which settled without treatment in 1 week.

Sideroblastic anaemia

A hypochromic anaemia with normal serum iron and total iron binding capacity raises the possibility of a sideroblastic anaemia. This is an anaemia due to defective blood formation in which ringed sideroblasts (nucleated red cell precursors containing iron granules arranged in a perinuclear ring) are formed in the marrow (Thomas and Powell, 1971). As far as the elderly are concerned there are two main types.

Primary acquired

This is a heterogeneous condition affecting the middle-aged and elderly in which a variety of deficiencies have been described (Cartwright and Deiss, 1975). In some cases there is a full or partial response to pyridoxine, which should be given in a dose of 100–1000 mg/day for several weeks. Deficiency of other haematinics, such as folic acid, may be present and should be corrected. Often the haemoglobin is maintained and no treatment is necessary but transfusion is sometimes needed. Repeated transfusions (and treatment with iron) will cause iron overload. Removing excess iron by venesection or desferrioxamine does not improve the anaemia (Dagg *et al.*, 1971).

Secondary

The haematological picture is similar to the primary acquired type but is caused by a variety of drugs and chronic illnesses. Some of the more important are:

(1) Drugs that interfere with pyridoxine metabolism (e.g. Isoniazid, PAS, cycloserine).
(2) Lead poisoning, alcoholism.

(3) Myeloma, rheumatoid arthritis, malabsorption and carcinomas.

Megaloblastic anaemia

B_{12} deficiency

This is the commonest cause of megaloblastic anaemia and has been found in 9% of anaemic and 5% of non-anaemic elderly subjects (McLennan *et al.*, 1973). The prevalence of known pernicious anaemia is about twice that of unrecognised cases.

The usual causes of B_{12} deficiency are pernicious anaemia, gastrectomy and malabsorption due to coeliac disease, but any disease that affects the terminal ileum may be responsible. Nutritional deficiency is rare, even in vegans.

Clinical features   Often the anaemia develops insidiously and the patient may have had shortness of breath and persistent ankle swelling for months before seeking medical advice. An acute infection may precipitate a crisis. Mental changes, mainly apathy, poor memory and depression are common and occasionally severe. The patient may in addition complain of loss of appetite and diarrhoea.

The association between B_{12} deficiency and dementia is far from being clear. Both are common and frequently coexist. Where mental changes are of recent onset and are associated with severe anaemia the prospects for recovery following B_{12} treatment are good. However long-standing dementia with only slight lowering of the serum B_{12} level is a poor therapeutic prospect. Mental changes, due to B_{12} deficiency, in the absence of anaemia, megaloblastic erythropoiesis or subacute combined degeneration of the cord were described in three patients by Strachan and Henderson (1965). All improved with B_{12} therapy. On the other hand, Hughes *et al.* (1970) found no evidence that B_{12} was superior to placebo in improving the wellbeing of elderly subjects with low serum B_{12} levels.

Neurological changes are usually a peripheral neuropathy with characteristic patchy anaesthesia, diminished reflexes and tender feet and calves. Rarely subacute combined degeneration of the cord, optic atrophy and cerebellar ataxia may occur.

Investigations   In addition to a low haemoglobin there is usually a raised mean corpuscular volume (over 100 $c\mu$) and a reduced platelet and white cell count. Bone marrow examination and a low serum B_{12} level confirm the diagnosis. It is not uncommon to find low normal serum B_{12} levels (i.e. 100–140 pg/100 ml in the absence of anaemia or megaloblasts, and it has been suggested that these patients have latent pernicious anaemia. The secretion of intrinsic factor is reduced and close follow-up is necessary to detect the first sign of frank B_{12} deficiency (Callender and Spray, 1962). Low serum B_{12} levels measured by the microbiological assay method can be an artifact resulting from the patient taking atibiotics. Deficiency of iron and folate should also be looked for and a Schilling test done to distinguish pernicious anaemia from intestinal malabsorption. Schilling tests are relatively expensive and of doubtful accuracy if the patient is incontinent and it has been argued that in the very elderly it is justifiable to simply ignore the test and start B_{12} therapy. One must be careful, if adopting this approach, not to miss other deficiencies due to malabsorption.

Immune phenomena   There are two types of antibody to intrinsic factor. The blocking antibody that prevents the combination of B_{12} with intrinsic factor is present in about 60% of patients with pernicious anaemia. The binding antibody prevents the attachment of intrinsic factor to the ileal mucosa and occurs in about 30%. The presence of intrinsic factor antibodies is a useful aid in diagnosis since they are rarely found in other disorders (Hoffbrand, 1971).

Parietal cell antibodies occur in about 90% of patients with pernicious anaemia. However the incidence in control subjects rises with age up to 16% in those over 60 years compared with 5% in those under 60 years. The incidence is also increased in relatives of patients with pernicious anaemia, in atrophic gastritis and achlorhydria, in thyrotoxicosis, myxoedema, chronic active hepatitis, rheumatoid arthritis, diabetes mellitus and iron deficiency anaemia.

Up to 40% of patients with pernicious anaemia may have antibodies to thyroid cytoplasm or thyroglobulin and they may respond to steroids.

Treatment Patients with severe anaemia (haemoglobin less than 5 g/100 ml) can die from heart failure before B_{12} therapy becomes effective and transfusion with packed cells is needed. Vitamin B_{12} is given in the form of hydroxocobalamin 1000 μg injections i.m. on alternate days for 2 weeks to correct the anaemia and replenish stores. Thereafter 500 μg every 3 months is sufficient and must be continued throughout life. Sudden death sometimes occurs during B_{12} therapy and has been attributed in the past to hypokalaemia; this is no longer thought to be the case and routine potassium supplements are unnecessary. Iron deficiency may develop, shown by a failure of haemoglobin to rise and a microcytosis: ferrous sulphate 200 mg twice daily will then be needed.

Folate deficiency

This can be due to malnutrition (see Chapter 9) malabsorption, excessive demands (such as malignancy, haemolytic anaemia or chronic inflammatory diseases) or drugs (e.g. anticonvulsants and trimethoprim). It is much less common than B_{12} deficiency as a cause of anaemia and in one series of 90 cases of megaloblastic anaemia only one was due to pure folate deficiency compared with 30 due to B_{12} deficiency (Evans *et al.*, 1968). However low folate was often found as part of a mixed deficiency, particularly associated with iron deficiency. A raised serum folate with a low serum B_{12} level can follow bacterial overgrowth in a stagnant loop of bowel.

Clinical features There is usually a mild anaemia which is normocytic in the early stages and later macrocytic. Mental changes are common, particularly apathy and confusion, and this often responds promptly to treatment. Dementia has been attributed to folate deficiency (Strachan and Henderson, 1967) which improved when the deficiency was corrected.

Investigations One difficulty is to decide which level of serum folate represents true folate deficiency. Levels below 6 ng are common in the elderly and were found by Read *et al.* (1965) in 80% of consecutive admissions to a residential home for the elderly. This figure dropped to 67% when grossly anaemic patients were excluded. A survey of the folate status in the elderly by Girdwood *et al.* (1967) concluded that since there was an overlap between folate deficient and normal subjects, a serum folate as low as 2.2 ng does not necessarily indicate folate deficiency. The serum folate fluctuates considerably with variations in diet and absorption, and measuring the red cell folate gives a more accurate picture of the tissue folate concentration. It is also a useful test when folate deficiency is thought of some time after the patient has been admitted to hospital, since it reflects the folate status over the previous 4 months. Red cell folate may be low in B_{12} deficiency (compared to a normal or high serum folate) and should not therefore be used as the sole measure of folate status. Once the diagnosis of folate deficiency is established it is necessary to consider the cause. A full dietary and drug history is essential and, if normal, tests for malabsorption are indicated.

Treatment   5 mg of folic acid a day for 3–4 months is sufficient to treat the deficit and replenish stores. Thereafter a regular maintenance dose will be needed in some patients with malabsorption or who continue with anticonvulsant therapy.

Other macrocytic anaemias

Hypothyroidism
There is an increased incidence of pernicious anaemia, but a macrocytic normoblastic anaemia due to thyroxine deficiency may occur as well as an iron deficiency anaemia.

Scurvy
Subclinical vitamin C deficiency is quite common in elderly men (see Chapter 9) and often coexists with other deficiencies. There is no direct correlation between vitamin C and haemoglobin levels and anaemia has been variously described as hypochromic (possibly due to blood loss) normochromic or macrocytic. The marrow may be normoblastic or megaloblastic. If there is a poor response to treatment

with vitamin C then folic acid or iron should be added, depending on the blood picture.

Haemolytic anaemia

This should be suspected where there is a rapidly falling haemoglobin with no sign of blood loss. There is a raised unconjugated bilirubin; serum iron and total iron binding capacity are increased; the reticulocyte count is above 2% and the marrow shows active red cell proliferation with increased iron stores. Intravascular haemolysis produces methaemalbumen in the plasma and this can be detected by Schumm's spectroscopic test. The haemolytic anaemias can be divided into congenital and acquired, and although hereditary spherocytic anaemia has been described in the elderly it is more usual to see haemolytic anaemia secondary to the presence of antibodies.

Primary acquired   Antibodies of either the warm or cold type may be found. Prednisone (40–60 mg/day) is the first line of treatment; transfusions should be avoided.

Secondary acquired   Some degree of haemolytic anaemia is common in leukaemia and other malignancies. Cold agglutinins may be found in polyarteritis nodosa and mycoplasma pneumonia. Drugs may have a direct toxic effect on red cells and cause haemolysis (e.g. phenacetin, phenylhydrazine). The direct Coombs test is usually negative. Hypersensitivity reactions to drugs (e.g. methyl dopa, penicillin, salicylates) also occur, though many patients have a positive direct Coombs reaction without actually developing haemolytic anaemia.

Anaemia of chronic disorders

In the elderly this is very common. It is usually mild and characterized by a low serum iron, low total binding capacity, decreased saturation of transferrin, decreased bone marrow sideroblasts and normal or increased reticuloendothelial iron (Cartwright and Lee, 1971). After the first month of the illness a balance is struck between red cell production and destruction and the degree of anaemia remains constant.

Blood disorders

The picture is usually normochromic and normocytic but may be normocytic and hypochromic or rarely, where disease is long-standing, hypochromic and microcytic. Although found in chronic infections it is often associated in the elderly with rheumatoid arthritis, malignancy, fractures, collagen diseases and chronic renal failure.

Treatment is directed towards the underlying cause. Transfusion is rarely indicated and iron therapy of no value except in some patients (particularly those with rheumatoid arthritis) who have iron deficiency shown by a low serum iron, normal total iron binding capacity and absent bone marrow iron.

Anaemia responsive to steroids

Anaemia, usually normochromic and normocytic, with a high ESR and dysproteinaemia (raised α_2 globulin) may be part of the cranial arteritis–polymyalgia syndrome. There is a rapid response to treatment with steroids.

CHRONIC LYMPHATIC LEUKAEMIA

This is mainly a disease of the elderly and typically presents insidiously with increasing fatigue, loss of appetite, palpable lymph nodes, recurrent infections or an attack of hepes zoster. The disease may be asymptomatic and discovered only on routine blood count. The course varies from: (1) a relatively benign form which, untreated, remains stationary for many years; (2) a similar course plus the complication of haemolytic anaemia or thrombocytopenia; (3) development of immunological abnormalities; to finally (4) an accelerated malignant phase. When deciding on treatment it is essential to consider the patient as a whole and to use powerful drugs with unpleasant side-effects only if the patient's condition warrants them.

Chlorambucil (0.2 mg/kg) may be given initially for 6 weeks and the dose reduced as the lymphocyte count falls and lymph node masses shrink. Anaemia and thrombocytopenia are not improved by chlorambucil but will usually respond well to prednisone 40 mg/day.

251

Radiotherapy will be needed for lymph nodes that are painful or causing pressure symptoms.

MULTIPLE MYELOMA

This is the commonest of the monoclonal gammopathies and increases in frequency with age. The sexes are equally affected.

TABLE 2

CLASSIFICATION OF MONOCLONAL GAMMOPATHIES
(After Alexanian, 1977)

Condition	Approximate frequency %
Plasma cell myelomas	
Multiple myeloma	
symptomatic	65
asymptomatic	2
Localized plasmacytoma	5
Waldenström's macroglobulinaemia	8
Heavy chain disease	1
Primary amyloidosis (without myeloma)	1
Benign type	20

Clinical features

The commonest presenting symptom is bone pain, usually from the spine or ribs. Pain developing after a trivial injury should arouse suspicion of a pathological fracture. Many patients complain only of weight loss and the non-specific symptoms attributable to anaemia. Recurrent chest infections due to impaired immunoglobulin production are a frequent feature. Occasionally the symptoms of hypercalcaemia (confusion, vomiting and constipation), root pain, spinal cord compression due to vertebral body collapse or renal failure predominate.

Investigations

The diagnosis of multiple myeloma is not always straightforward since any of the recognized laboratory or X-ray criteria may be negative in a particular patient. The following are the most important features:

Osteolytic bone lesions
These are seen most often in the spine, pelvis, skull and ribs and tend to be more clearly defined than the lesions produced by metastases from a carcinoma of the bronchus, breast, kidney or thyroid. In contrast to patients with bony metastases over 85% of those with myeloma have a normal alkaline phosphatase. Generalized demineralization of vertebral bodies must be distinguished from osteoporosis.

Plasma proteins
The total level of proteins is usually raised, and in 95% of patients electrophoresis will demonstrate an abnormal monoclonal protein. In about half the patients this will be IgG and in a quarter IgA. IgD, IgM and IgE paraproteins are rare.

Bence Jones protein
Normally only very small amounts of immunoglobulin light chains are excreted in the urine and these contain both K and L proteins. In myeloma, not only is the amount considerably increased but it is of one type only, K or L. Bence Jones protein is present in about 50% of patients with myeloma but may also be found in Waldenström's macroglobulinaemia and in cases of carcinoma with bony secondaries.

Plasmacystosis
Examination of the bone marrow shows an increase in abnormal plasma cells. The number of cells is not a prognostic guide.

Blood film
Usually there is a normocytic, normochromic anaemia secondary to malignancy, renal failure or bone infiltration. Occasionally there may

be a hypochromic, macrocytic or leuko-erythroblastic picture. Rouleaux formation of red cells can sometimes be seen.

ESR
This is raised, often above 100 mm/h, in over 90% of patients.

Hypercalcaemia
A serum calcium greater than 2.68 mmol/l (11.5 g/100 ml) is found in about one-third of patients.

Renal failure
This is usually associated with the passage of large amounts of Bence Jones protein, but may be due to hypercalcaemia, hyperuricaemia or amyloidosis.

The prognosis is poorer in the very elderly and those with a large tumour mass indicated by: (1) haemoglobin less than 8.5 g/100 ml; (2) calcium $>$ 2.68 mmol/l; (3) serum IgG peak $>$ 70 g/l; (4) extensive lytic lesions (Alexanian, 1977).

Management

As with chronic lymphatic leukaemia not all patients need chemotherapy. When they do, however, it is best handled, including close follow-up to detect early relapse, by a specialist centre. Intermittent 4-day courses of melphelan and prednisone repeated at 4-week intervals is currently the initial treatment of choice. Cyclophosphamide is as good as, but not superior to, melphelan. Additional physical and moral support is essential. Radiotherapy will do much to relieve bone pain and spinal cord compression. Long bones, particularly around the neck of the femur, that are severely lysed and look to be in danger of breaking are more easily fixed by an orthopaedic surgeon before a fracture rather than afterwards.

The patient should be encouraged to drink plenty of fluids if hyperviscosity (monoclonal protein $>$ 50 g/l, spontaneous haemorrhages, papilloedema, loss of vision, fatigue) or hypercalcaemia are a problem. Dehydration prior to an i.v. pyelogram is a well recognized hazard and the contrast medium (iodipamide) used in i.v. cholangiograms can precipitate Bence Jones protein and cause renal failure. Hypercalaemia persisting despite treatment with diuretics and steroids is an indication for melphelan. Severe anaemia will require transfusion of packed cells. The patient should be kept mobile as much as pain allows; analgesics will be needed and a corset may be helpful.

WALDENSTRÖM'S MACROGLOBULINAEMIA

This is a rare, chronic, lymphoproliferative disorder that is seen most often in elderly men. The patient presents with weight loss, fatigue and recurrent infections. Hepatosplenomegaly, lymphadenopathy, anaemia and a raised ESR are typical. There is always a monoclonal gammopathy of IgM type and, in about 10% of patients, Bence Jones protein. Management is along similar lines to that of multiple myeloma.

BENIGN MONOCLONAL GAMMOPATHY

About 1% of the general population, rising to 6% in those over 80 years, are affected. An M-band is present but in contrast to multiple myeloma or macroglobulinaemia the concentration is usually low (< 20 g/l) and does not increase with time. There are no signs or symptoms of disease, ESR and haemoglobin remain steady and limited follow-up shows no progression (Axelsson and Hällén, 1968). However it is now thought that if the patient lives long enough multiple myeloma supervenes and continued surveillance is recommended.

POLYCYTHAEMIA

Primary

This is one of the myeloproliferative disorders and is most common in middle and late life. Symptoms can be non-specific and consist of weakness, dizziness and tiredness, or there may be signs and symptoms of a cerebral thrombosis, myocardial infarct or peripheral vascular disease. The patient is plethoric with peripheral cyanosis and the spleen may just be palpable. Haemoglobin is raised to 20 g/100 ml or more, the PCV to between 50 and 75% and the marrow shows proliferation of red cells. Treatment is by radioactive phosphorus (^{32}P). Acute leukaemia can result but the risk of it developing during the remaining life of an elderly person is low.

Secondary

As in the primary type the patient will be plethoric but the leukocyte count is normal and when due to hypoxia, clubbing and low arterial oxygen saturation will be present.

Hypoxia (commonly due to chronic bronchitis or acquired heart disease) is the major cause but polycythaemia may also be seen in renal carcinoma, polycystic kidney disease and cerebellar haemangioblastoma.

REFERENCES

Alexanian, R. (1978). Plasma cell neoplasms. *Medicine*, 2nd Series, **30** 1700

Axelsson, U. and Hällén, J. (1968). Review of fifty four subjects with monoclonal gammopathy. *Br. J. Haematol.*, **15**, 417

Beveridge, B. R., Bannerman, R. M., Evanson, J. M. and Witts, L. J. (1965). Hypochromic anaemia. *Q. J. Med.*, **34**, 145

Callender, S. T. and Spray, G. H. (1962). Latent pernicious anaemia. *Br. J. Haematol.*, **8**, 230

Cartwright, G. E. and Lee, G. R. (1971). The anaemia of chronic disorder. *Br. J. Haematol.*, **21**, 147

Cartwright, G. E. and Deiss, A. (1975). Sideroblasts, siderocytes and sideroblastic anaemia. *N. Engl. J. Med.*, **292**, 185

Dagg, J. H., Goldberg, A., Gibbs, W. N. and Anderson, J. R. (1966). Detection of latent pernicious anaemia in iron deficiency anaemia. *Br. Med. J.*, **2**, 619

Blood disorders

Dagg, J.H., Cumming, R. L. C. and Goldbert, A. (1971). Disorders of iron metabolism. In A. Goldberg and M. C. Brain (eds.). *Recent Advances in Haematology*. (Edingurgh: Churchill Livingstone)

Evans, D. M. D., Pathy, M. S., Sanerkin, N. G. and Deeble, T. J. (1968). Anaemia in geriatric patients. *Gerontol. Clin.*, **10,** 228

Girwood, R. H., Thomson, A. D. and Williamson, J. (1967). Folate status in the elderly. *Br. Med. J.*, **2,** 670

Hallberg, L. and Hogdahl, A. M. (1971). Anaemia and old age. *Gerontol. Clin.*, **13,** 31

Hoffbrand, A. V. (1971). The megaloblastic anaemias. In A. Goldberg and M. C. Brain (eds.). *Recent Advances in Haematology*. (Edinburgh: Churchill Livingstone)

Hughes, D., Elwood, P. C., Shinton, N. K. and Wrighton, R. J. (1970). Clinical trial of the effect of vitamin B_{12} in elderly subjects with low serum B_{12} levels. *Br. Med. J.*, **2,** 458

McLennan, W. J., Andrews, G. R., MacLeod, C. and Caird, F. I. (1973). Anaemia in the elderly. *Q. J. Med.* N.S., **42,** 1

Parsons, P. L., Withey, J. L. and Kilpatrick, G. S. (1965). The prevalence of anaemia in the elderly. *Practitioner,* **195,** 656

Read, A. E., Gough, K. R., Pardoe, J. L. and Nicholas, A. (1965). Nutritional studies on the entrants to an old people's home, with particular reference to folic acid deficiency. *Br. Med. J.*, **2,** 843

Strachan, R. W. and Henderson, J. G. (1965). Psychiatric syndromes due to avitaminosis B_{12} with normal blood and marrow. *Q.J.Med.*, N.S., **34,** 303

Strachan, R. W. and Henderson, J. G. (1967). Dementia and folate deficiency. *Q. J. Med.*, N.S., **36,** 189

Thomas, J. H. and Powell, D. E. B. (1971). *Blood Disorders in the Elderly*. (Bristol: John Wright and Sons)

Wright, W. B. (1967). Iron deficiency anaemia of the elderly treated by total dose infusion. *Gerontol. Clin.*, **9,** 107

257

13
Skin diseases

Along with connective tissue changes elsewhere in the body there is degeneration of dermal collagen with subsequent thinning and loss of elasticity of the skin. Environmental factors such as sun and wind are as important as ageing itself in causing wrinkling and roughening of the exposed skin. The skin is drier due to atrophy of eccrine and apocrine sweat glands and reduced sebum excretion. Pigmentary changes are common and may be isolated or widespread, particularly over exposed areas. In addition to male pattern baldness there is, in both sexes, a loss of hair follicles with diffuse thinning of hair.

Benign lesions that commonly appear with age include the following:

Senile purpura

These usually appear on the forearm or the back of the hand. They are caused by rupture of small blood vessels that have lost their network of collagen fibre support and become susceptible to trivial shearing injury.

259

Geriatrics

Seborrhoeic warts (benign basal cell papillomata)

These are yellowish, greasy plaques that become darker as they enlarge. They are most common on the trunk and scalp and are easily removed by curettage under local anaesthesia.

Campbell de Morgan spots

These are small, benign haemangiomata that are usually seen on the chest, abdomen, and upper limbs.

Senile lentigo

These are sometimes known as 'liver spots'. They are hyperpigmented macules that appear on sun-exposed areas, particularly the backs of the hands.

Onychogryphosis

This is hypertrophy with deformity of the nail plate. Initially the nails look heaped up but later become hard and clawlike. It may be caused by failure to cut the nails frequently, trauma, peripheral neuropathy or peripheral vascular disease.

SOME COMMON SKIN DISORDERS

Eczema

This is an inflammatory condition characterized by erythema, oedema, vesicles and itching. Atopic eczema is less common in the older patient and the more frequently encountered varieties are contact dermatitis and gravitational eczema.

Contact dermatitis
The dry skin of the elderly patient predisposes to sensitization, and although initially only the small area of skin exposed to the allergen is affected it may rapidly become widespread. Topical antibiotics or antihistamines, lanolin and a number of soaps, metals, household

260

cleaners and plants can be responsible. Patch testing is needed to confirm the diagnosis. Treatment involves avoiding the allergen, topical steroids and an oral antihistamine.

Gravitational eczema

Long-standing leg oedema, from any cause, is likely to be complicated by eczema and lichenification. A secondary rash may spread over the thighs, abdomen and arms. Topical antibiotics should be avoided because of the risk of sensitization. The feet should be elevated to reduce oedema and Lassar's paste with 15% glycerin applied to the affected area and covered by an elasto-crepe bandage (Verbov, 1974).

Intertrigo

There is a well-marked area of inflammation with a scallop edge that typically occurs in moist areas such as the groin or beneath pendulous breasts. Regular washing and use of talcum powder will control mild cases but where there is severe bacterial or candidal infection a steroid cream containing an antibiotic and antifungal agent (e.g. TriAdcortyl) gives very good results.

Herpes zoster

Elderly, frail patients with an underlying malignancy are especially susceptible. The main problem is post-herpetic neuralgia which can be severe and may persist for 6 months or more. The risk of this complication is considerably reduced by the use of idoxuridine. The rash should be covered in gauze soaked with 40% idoxuridine in dimethyl sulphoxide (DMSO) and rewetted daily for 3 or 4 days until the vesicles dry (Juel-Jensen, 1973). Idoxuridine in that strength or in DMSO cannot be used on mucosal surfaces and advice on treatment of herpes involving the eyes should be obtained from an ophthalmologist.

Severe herpes zoster may merit intravenous cytosine arabinoside (*Br.Med.J.* Leader, 1976). Systemic corticosteroids do not influence healing time or the early pain of zoster but they do shorten the duration of post-herpetic neuralgia and are considered safe (Eaglstein *et al.*, 1970). Prednisone 60 mg a day may be given for a week from the first appearance of the rash. Relief of post-herpetic neuralgia may be obtained from analgesics and tranquillizers and gentle massage over the affected area with a vibrator.

Bullous pemphigoid

Although confined mainly to the elderly it is still uncommonly seen. Large, tense, subepidermal bullae appear on the limbs and lower abdomen. They do not itch. Other blistering conditions from which it must be distinguished include skin infections, oedema, contact dermatitis, the idiopathic blistering that may occur on a paralysed limb following a stroke and pemphigus. It is an autoimmune disease, benign and self-limiting compared with pemphigus. Control is rapidly achieved with prednisone 40–60 mg daily.

Basal cell carcinoma (rodent ulcer)

This is the commonest of the skin malignancies and usually appears as a nodule with a shiny raised edge. There may be ulceration with a crust that bleeds easily if broken. It grows slowly, rarely metastasizes and usually appears on the upper face, scalp, trunk and arms. Other presentations include the morphea-like (yellowish, slightly raised) plaque and chronic superficial patches of dry, scaly erythema. Treatment is by excision or radiotherapy.

Squamous cell carcinoma

Sun exposure, leukoplakia or previous damage to the skin are predisposing factors, but it can appear anywhere on the skin or mucous membranes. It is a true invasive tumour that usually begins as a hard nodule and may ulcerate or grow warty or papillomatous. There is a surrounding area of induration and metastases are common. Excision is best but radiotherapy is effective for small lesions.

Malignant melanoma

This can occur at any age and carries a poor prognosis. Typically there is a blue-black nodule that increases in size although any lesion that ulcerates or bleeds should arouse suspicion. The amelanotic type presenting as a granulomatous nodule, often on the sole of the foot, is easily missed. Wide excision of the lesion and involved lymph nodes is required.

Kerato-acanthoma (Molluscum sebaceum)

This is a benign tumour that grows more rapidly than a basal cell carcinoma and reaches its full size in a few weeks. It is a firm nodule containing a central crater with a keratin plug. It clears up spontaneously within about 6 months leaving a shallow scar. It is best removed by curettage followed by cauterization.

Pruritis

Because of the tendency towards dryness it is common for the elderly to complain of pruritis in cold weather, if they live in centrally heated surroundings or if they bathe too frequently. Other causes that should be looked for include:

(1) Skin diseases such as eczema, psoriasis or lichen planus.
(2) Scabies and other infestations.
(3) Obstructive jaundice.
(4) Anaemia.
(5) Endocrine – diabetes mellitus, hypo- and hyper-thyroidism.
(6) Malignancies.
(7) Uraemia.
(8) Drug reactions.

Patients with a dry skin should avoid soap and use ung. emulsificans instead. Aqueous cream and an oral antihistamine such as trimeprazine may help; 1% hydrocortisone cream is useful if the itching is severe.

LEG ULCERS

Venous

Of the several types of leg ulcer this is by far the commonest. The condition depends on deep vein incompetence which is usually secondary to thrombosis. Ankle oedema develops, the amount depending on how much time the patient spends sitting down with his feet dependent and the presence or absence of congestive heart failure. Red, scaly, itchy patches of dermatitis appear, pigmentation is common and, either due to scratching or to some other trauma, an ulcer develops. It is always on the lower half of the leg, most commonly over the medial malleolus, and has soft irregular edges.

Because of the danger of eczematous reactions, it is best to avoid applying topical antibiotics. Steroids are unhelpful unless there is a considerable local inflammation. The mainstay of treatment is to apply, from the toes to above the knee, a firm elastic 'blue line' bandage and to combine with this exercises designed to increase venous blood flow. Oedema delays healing and the patient should walk as much as possible, avoid standing and sit with feet up on a stool. If the ulcer is infected it should be cleaned with a half-strength eusol solution or the slough removed with Debrisan. When the ulcer is clean the leg should be covered from toes to knee with an occlusive Viscopaste bandage, which is left in place for 2 weeks between changes and allows uninterrupted healing. With large ulcers, once they are clean and free from streptococcal infection, pigskin grafting should be tried since the results are often very satisfactory.

Treatments designed for venous ulcers are legion and it should be remembered that, regardless of the technique, success is directly proportional to the enthusiasm and persistence of the medical and nursing staff.

Arterial

These are usually much more painful than venous ulcers. They tend to be smaller and affect the toes and anterior part of the leg (see Peripheral vascular disease, p. 135).

Skin diseases

Miscellaneous

Leg ulcers in diabetics may be arterial or neuropathic. Small, painful ulcers are seen on the foot and anterior part of the leg in collagen diseases. Leg ulcers may complicate rheumatoid disease and ulcerative colitis.

Trauma to the skin of an elderly person (particularly a V-shaped wound) can result in a very slowly healing ulcer. Initial suturing under tension aggravates the difficulties of poor blood supply and venous drainage and should be avoided. It is best to simply apply adhesive skin sutures, avoiding any tension, and cover with unmedicated tulle gras and a Viscopaste bandage from the toes to below the knee. The Viscopaste is changed every 2 weeks until the wound is healed (*Br.Med.J.*, Leader, 1978).

PRESSURE SORES

The basic lesion is ischaemic due to prolonged pressure on the skin. Reduction or obstruction to blood flow follows when the average capillary pressure is greater than 25–30 mmHg. Poor mobility, loss of subcutaneous fat and maceration of skin due to soiling with urine or faeces are predisposing factors. Discomfort following lying or sitting in one posture is a stimulus to change position but the unconscious or weakened patient may be unable to move without help. The importance of spontaneous bodily movements in preventing pressure sores was shown by Exton-Smith and Sherwin (1961). Using a specially designed apparatus that recorded changes in bodily position at night they found that the incidence of pressure sores was directly related to the number of spontaneous movements made during sleep. Patients with high mobility scores needed no special nursing, but those whose scores were low, or who showed a rapidly falling score in successive nights, were very liable to pressure sores and required active prophylaxis.

Clinical experience shows that the general condition of the patient is of great importance in determining whether or not a pressure sore will develop. Use of a simple scoring system (see Table 1), with a maximum of 20 points for the patient in good physical condition and a minimum of 5 points for one in a very poor physical state, correlates closely with the incidence of pressure sores. Thus almost 50% of patients who initially scored less than 12 developed pressure sores compared with 5% who scored between 18 and 20 (Norton, McLaren and Exton-Smith, 1975). Sores are particularly likely to develop

TABLE 1
RISK OF DEVELOPING PRESSURE SORES

A. General Physical Condition	B. Mental	C. Activity	D. Mobility	E. Incontinence
4 Good	4 Alert	4 Ambulant	4 Full	4 Not
3 Fair	3 Apathetic	3 Walks/help	3 Slightly limited	3 Occasional
2 Poor	2 Confused	2 Chairbound	2 Very limited	2 Usually/urine
1 Very bad	1 Stupor	1 Bed	1 Immobile	1 Doubly

over bony prominences such as the heels, hips, sacrum and shoulder-blades. The shearing stress, when a patient slips down the bed from a sitting position, especially affects those areas and causes rupture of blood vessels and tissue necrosis. It has been suggested that an important contribution to tissue necrosis is the accumulation of anaerobic metabolic waste products due to occlusion of the lymph vessels (Krouskop *et al.*, 1978).

Necrosis begins first in fat and muscle and a developing sore may appear only as skin which is slightly reddened and has a boggy feel to it. At this stage a sore can be prevented if the pressure is relieved. If neglected the skin blisters and sloughs, and although only a small patch may appear to be involved the area of necrosis hidden from view

266

spreads out widely and deeply. Osteomyelitis may be a complication and the loss of blood and protein-rich serous fluid causes serious debility.

Prophylaxis

Prevention of pressure sores is the hallmark of adequate numbers of skilled nurses. However, many patients develop a sore before admission to hospital, particularly those who have fallen, fractured the femoral neck and lain all night on the floor. A double-blind trial on patients undergoing surgery to the hip and upper femur found that a single dose of ACTH gel (80 i.u.) given pre-operatively effectively reduced the incidence of sores (Barton and Barton, 1976). In animals it has been shown that ACTH administered 4 hours before trauma stabilizes the endothelial cell junctions and prevents separation. The timing of the injection is crucial since it must be given before the endothelial cell separation begins to occur. This is possible in elective hip surgery but not always for patients with a fractured neck of femur who may not be seen until long after the damage is done.

Various types of bed have been designed to relieve pressure on vulnerable points. In a controlled trial a large-celled ripple mattress was found to be superior to an ordinary hospital mattress in preventing and healing pressure sores of the trunk and heels, and appeared to afford protection to patients in whatever position they might be lying (Bliss, McLaren and Exton-Smith, 1967). The conclusion of another trial was that the two systems which produced pressure consistently lower than capillary pressure were: (1) the low air loss patient support system (Watkins & Watson Ltd., London), which consists of a mobile air support system (covered by a fabric permeable to water vapour) on which the patient is supported by a continuous flow of temperature-controlled air at pressures below 20 mmHg.; and (2) a bed of freshly shaken feather pillows (at least eight) on a foam base (Redfern *et al.*, 1973). It must be emphasized that no mattress in itself will prevent sores unless, in addition, the patient is regularly turned.

Management

Treatment of the established sore consists mainly of cleaning and packing with dressings soaked in half-strength Eusol. Keeping the skin dry and free from urine and faeces and use of a silicon-based cream such as Dimethicone are also important. Ultraviolet light and infrared treatment help to clean the sore and promote healing. Applications of white of egg, or insulin dried off with oxygen, are among the many methods which have been tried, but it appears to matter little which exotic treatment is used so long as the nurse is encouraged to apply it at frequent intervals.

Iron and vitamin supplements may be needed and a blood transfusion often produces a considerable improvement in a debilitated patient. Zinc supplements do not accelerate healing unless it can be shown that there is depletion (*Lancet* Leader, 1973). Sheepskin protectors for the heels, a bed cradle to lift the blankets off the feet, an air cushion for the chair and 'bean bag' chairs that mould themselves to the patient's shape are all useful aids.

REFERENCES

Barton, A. A. and Barton, M. (1976). Drug-based prevention of pressure-sores. *Lancet*, **ii**, 443

Bliss, M. R., McLaren, R. and Exton-Smith, A. N. (1967). Preventing pressure sores in hospital: controlled trial of a large-celled ripple mattress, *Br. Med. J.*, **1**, 394

Eaglstein, W. H., Katz, R. and Brown, J. A. (1970). The effects of early corticosteroid therapy on the skin eruption and pain of herpes zoster. *J. Am. Med. Assoc.*, **211**, 1681

Exton-Smith, A. N. and Sherwin, R. W. (1961). The prevention of pressure sores: significance of spontaneous bodily movements. *Lancet*, **ii**, 1124

Juel-Jensen, B. E. (1973). The chemotherapy of viral diseases, *Br. J. Hosp. Med.*, **10**, 402

Krouskop, T. A., Reddy, N. P., Spencer, W. A. and Secor, J. W. (1978). Mechanism of decubitus ulcer formation – an hypothesis, *Med. Hypoth.*, **4**, 37

Skin diseases

Leader (1973). Zinc deficiency in man. *Lancet*, **i,** 299

Leader (1976). Chemotherapy for varicella – zoster infections, *Br. Med. J.*, **2,** 1466

Leader (1978), Flap lacerations. *Br. Med. J.*, **1,** 4

Norton, D., McLaren, R. and Exton-Smith, A. N. (1975). *An Investigation of Geriatric Nursing Problems in Hospital*, 1st reprint. (Edinburgh: Churchill Livingstone)

Redfern, S. J., Jeneid, P. A., Gillingham, M. E. and Fletcher Lunn, H. (1973). Local pressures with ten types of patient-support systems, *Lancet*, **ii,** 277

Verbov, J. (1974). *Skin Diseases in the Elderly*. (London: William Heinemann)

14
The musculoskeletal system

I. BONE DISEASE

AGEING IN BONE

Ageing is accompanied by loss of bone from the skeleton; the atrophy of bone corresponds to atrophy of other tissues which occurs with increasing age.

The most comprehensive data of the effects of ageing in the skeleton have been derived from morphometric studies. In a simple technique the length (L) of the bone (usually the second metacarpal) on a hand radiograph is measured with a millimetre rule and at the midpoint the diameter of the medullary canal (d) and the periosteal envelope (D) are measured with a vernier caliper. The transverse cross-sectional cortical area of the second metacarpal, calculated from measurements of X-rays, correlates well with the ash content as determined by incineration (Gryfe, Exton-Smith and Stewart, 1972).

Various derived formulae, such as the ratio of cortical area to total area $(D^2 - d^2)/D^2$ and the ratio of cortical area to surface area $(D^2 - d^2)/DL$, have been used to correct for differing skeletal size between individuals.

Using the ratio cortical area/surface area percentile ranking curves

271

for the normal population of men and women between the ages of 2 and 85 years have been constructed (Exton-Smith *et al.*, 1969; Gryfe *et al.*, 1971) (see figure 1, p. 283).

The features of bone development and loss as revealed by these curves are:

(a) The curves for the percentile ranks (10, 25, 50, 75 and 90) remain roughly parallel with age; that is, the variance remains unchanged with age and the distribution at each age group is normal.

(b) There is a rapid increase in the amount of bone during the period of growth (up to the age of 17), but the increase continues at a slower rate for another 12 years or so after increase in height has ceased.

(c) Loss of bone is steady after about the age of 45, occurring more rapidly in women than in men.

(d) There are some individuals aged 80 who have more bone than others at the age of 30.

OSTEOPOROSIS

The classical definition of osteoporosis by Albright is 'too little bone, but what bone there is, is normal'. Osteoporosis has characteristic clinical, radiological and pathological features which can usually distinguish it from other forms of metabolic bone disease. It is the end-result of a number of processes which lead to a diminution in the amount of bone in the skeleton.

Aetiology

Some of the important factors influencing the amount of bone in old age include the skeletal status at maturity, the loss of bone with age in later life in both sexes, and the more rapid bone loss following the menopause in women. Thus those individuals who have densely calcified bones at maturity may be at an advantage; the skeleton will remain adequate even when, in later life, part of the bone material is lost.

Postmenopausal bone loss
There is a rapid bone loss during the first 10 years after the menopause. The administration of oestrogens (Davis *et al.*, 1966) prevents this initial rapid loss; but loss still continues at a slower rate with the curves parallel at a higher level.

Immobilization
Immobility due to fracture, joint disease, splinting and hemiplegia leads to localized osteoporosis. Generalized osteoporosis due to immobilization may complicate other forms and initiate a vicious circle. In particular, many old people, mainly women, become largely sedentary, a situation almost certainly to blame in part for their frequent osteoporosis.

Hyperadrenocorticism
Osteoporosis is a well-known clinical feature in patients with Cushing's syndrome. It also develops in patients treated for a number of years with corticosteroids for rheumatoid arthritis, asthma and skin diseases.

Calcium deficiency
Nordin (1971) has shown that the fasting urinary calcium of postmenopausal women is raised, and that the overnight or early morning excretion of calcium exceeds the amount that can be stored during the day. The increased bone resorption in the fasting state is attributed to the loss of the protective action of oestrogens against parathyroid hormone.

Vitamin D deficiency
A further factor in senile osteoporosis may be a fall in calcium absorption which occurs in men and women after the age of 70. In part impaired calcium absorption may be due to vitamin D deficiency which is not uncommon in the elderly, especially women. In the majority of cases the vitamin D deficiency is not detected until severe

enough to cause osteomalacia. Correction of the deficiency promotes the absorption of calcium.

Fluoride
Some epidemiological studies have shown that osteoporosis is more common in older people living in areas with a low content of fluoride in the water supply. This finding has not been confirmed by differences in the incidence of osteoporosis in the high-fluoride area of West Hartlepool compared with the low-fluoride area of Leeds. It is possible that the influence of fluoride is exerted only during the period of bone growth in childhood rather than in adult life; that is, the action of fluoride, like that of other nutrients, in the prevention of osteoporosis in old age may be exerted maximally in the first 20 years of life.

Gastrectomy
Histological section reveals that following gastrectomy there is an excessive amount of thin osteoid seams, whereas in simple osteoporosis osteoid seams are absent. The distinctive findings in post-gastrectomy cases are considered to be due to calcium deficiency. Gastrectomy appears to accelerate the effects of ageing on loss of bone from the skeleton.

Clinical features

The symptoms range from no complaint at all to attacks of severe backache which may be completely disabling. The backache may be precipitated by muscular effort, e.g. turning the trunk in reaching to lift an object from a wall shelf, and this points to collapse of a vertebral body which is subsequently revealed on X-ray examination. The pain may last a few weeks followed by a period of up to 10 or more years in which the pain is completely absent. The pain is felt in the back occasionally radiating to the buttocks and down the legs. It is usually relieved by immobilization and made much worse by movement — patients often remark that it is worse when they try to turn their position in bed at night. Wedging of the mid-thoracic vertebrae occurs early in the course of the disease and produces the dowager's hump deformity; this is later followed by spontaneous crush fractures of the dorsilumbar region. The collapse fractures lead to progressive incremental loss of height. The lower ribs in severe cases often override the iliac crests. A transverse band of keratinized skin appears over the upper abdomen. This is highly suggestive of osteoporosis and is rarely present in other conditions causing vertebral collapse.

Radiology

Increased translucency of bone is the main feature. This affects all bones, but trabecular bone in the spine appears relatively more affected. The vertebral bodies appear hollow, outlined by the shell of cortical bone. Impaction fractures of the brittle bones occur, affecting the mid-thoracic vertebrae; but the vertebral bodies are not uniformly involved so that some retain their shape with collapsed vertebrae intervening. The bodies of the lumbar vertebrae become biconcave due to the expansion into them of the intervertebral discs. Sometimes localized protrusions of the nucleus pulposus occur giving rise to Schmorl's nodes. Although biconcavity in the lumbar region is the typical appearance and is seen in very old people it can only occur at a stage when the disc is fluid and capable of expansion. But, as the disc becomes rigid with advancing age, the lumbar vertebral bodies may become wedged similar to the thoracic vertebrae. In the long bones diminution in cortical thickness is the salient feature; this is mainly the result of endosteal absorption.

Biochemistry

The serum calcium, inorganic phosphorus and alkaline phosphatase are normal in osteoporosis. Sometimes a moderate rise in the serum alkaline phosphatase occurs following fractures; even a small fracture can induce a temporary elevation lasting several weeks. When active absorption is occurring there is usually a slight increase in urinary calcium excretion.

Treatment

One of the chief difficulties in assessing the results of treatment is the episodic nature of the disorder and the fact that the acute episodes characterized by crush fractures are self-limiting. Thus, when the patient seeks treatment for the sudden onset of backache, spontaneous remission occurs within a few weeks irrespective of what drug therapy is given. It is important to avoid immobilization, which can only aggravate loss of bone. During an acute phase some patients gain confidence from the temporary use of a lumbar sacral elastic support, and at the same time are encouraged to remain active by walking with a stick.

The most effective treatment is that advocated by Albright, who showed that the use of sex hormones will reduce negative nitrogen and calcium balance. Stilboestrol (1–3 mg) or dienoestrol (0·3–0·9 mg) are given daily in courses of 4–5 weeks with 1 week's gap in between. Patients should be warned that withdrawal bleeding may occur after each course. Such a regimen reduces the incidence of fractures and leads to a cessation in the loss of height. A high calcium intake often produces a strikingly positive calcium balance. Moderate doses of vitamin D (100 i.u. daily) are advisable, since intakes are low for many old people, especially the housebound. In none of these methods of treatment has a convincing increase in bone density been demonstrated; indeed this may not be possible since new bone cannot be laid down where the old framework has disappeared. Jowsey et al. (1972) have recently evaluated in patients with osteoporosis the effects of fluoride administration combined with vitamin D and calcium. The optimum regimen was found to be 50 mg sodium fluoride and 900 mg supplemental calcium per day and 50 000 i.u. vitamin D twice a week. Eleven patients with progressive osteoporosis which was of sufficient severity to cause deformity of the vertebral bodies were treated for a period of at least one year. In all but one patient bone formation was increased after treatment, as assessed by examination of the iliac crest biopsy specimens. Although the newly formed bone is histologically normal in appearance it may be abnormally fragile and this treatment may have no influence on the subsequent fracture rate.

OSTEOMALACIA

Osteomalacia is a generalized disease of bone characterized by deficient calcification of a normal bone matrix. Histological examination reveals an increase in the amount of osteoid, that is, non-calcified matrix around the bone trabeculae. It is a disease produced by lack of vitamin D.

Prevalence in old age

Osteomalacia is not confined to any age group, but in old age there are many conditions which can give rise to it; consequently it is not uncommon. Anderson and his colleagues (1966) in Glasgow investigated a group of 100 women aged 68–93 years who had been newly admitted to a geriatric department and who had a possible clinical indication of osteomalacia (see Table 1). In this group 16 cases of osteomalacia were discovered. Subsequently 100 consecutive patients

TABLE 1
POSSIBLE CLINICAL INDICATIONS FOR OSTEOMALACIA

Vague and generalized pain	Bone tenderness
Low backache	Malabsorption states
Muscle weakness and stiffness	Long confinement indoors
Waddling gait	Malnutrition
Skeletal deformity	

admitted to the female wards were investigated and the incidence of osteomalacia was shown to be 4% of elderly women admitted to this geriatric department. Chalmers (1967), an orthopaedic surgeon in Edinburgh, and his colleagues have described the clinical features of 37 recently recognized cases of osteomalacia. Thirty-four of the 37 cases were women; their ages ranged from 39 to 89 years and the majority of patients were over the age of 70. They consider that osteomalacia is not uncommon in elderly women among whom it is likely to be confused with senile osteoporosis, and that there is a need for a

277

thorough screening of all elderly patients presenting with weakness, skeletal pain, pathological fractures or with diminished radiographic density of bone.

Aetiology

There are many causes of osteomalacia in old age and often the condition is caused by several factors coexisting in the same individual.

The main causes include inadequate dietary intake of vitamin D, lack of exposure to sunlight, malabsorption, gastrectomy, impaired hydroxylation of cholecalciferol in the liver and reduced conversion of 25-hydroxycholecalciferol to the active 1,25-dihydroxycholecalciferol due to impairment of renal function. The sources, absorption, metabolism and utilization of vitamin D are discussed in Chapter 9.

Clinical features

In the early stages the disease is often missed altogether because the bodily pains are thought to be due to 'rheumatism'. Owing to the poor localization of the pain, attention may not be directly focused on the bones. Later, pain is nagging, persistent and unremitting and it results from strain on tender soft bone, rather than fracture of non-tender brittle bone as in osteoporosis. In some cases the pain is very severe, even breathing becomes difficult and the weight of bedclothes pressing upon the ribs becomes unbearable.

Muscular weakness is often striking. This has been regarded as a typical feature of rickets for many years but it is only recently that the frequent occurrence of muscle weakness in osteomalacia has been recognized. It takes the form of a proximal myopathy. The patient may complain of difficulty in climbing stairs or getting up from a chair or difficulty in lifting the feet from the ground when walking, and this leads to a typical 'waddling gait'. It the shoulder girdle is involved the patient may be unable to brush her hair.

The patient becomes shorter owing to deformities of the trunk — usually kyphosis but less often scoliosis. The softening of the bones leads to angulation of the sternum, deformities of the pelvis and

278

bending of the femoral necks. Finally, on account of painful movements and skeletal deformities, the patient is forced to her bed.

Radiography

There is diminished radiographic density of bone and deformities may occur in the softened bone. Thus the pelvic brim may become bent as the result of the inward pressure of the femoral heads. The intervertebral discs are often ballooned and the soft vertebral bodies become biconvave in shape ('cod-fish vertebra'). Although typically the vertebral bodies are evenly involved in osteomalacia coexistent osteoporosis is so often present that there is an irregular distribution of crush fractures. Thus this point of distinction from osteoporosis, although useful in younger patients, is less reliable in old age.

A characteristic finding is the appearance of Looser's zones or pseudo-fractures. These are bands of decalcification perpendicular or oblique to the surface of the bone. The common sites are the axillary border of the scapula, the pubic rami, the ribs, the neck of the humerus and near the lesser trochanter of the femoral neck. They occur only in osteomalacia and when present make a certain differentiation from osteoporosis.

Sometimes the bone changes of secondary hyperparathyroidism are present with, for example, the appearance of subperiosteal erosions in the metacarpals or phalanges.

Biochemistry

The typical biochemical findings are a low or normal serum calcium, low serum inorganic phosphorus, raised serum alkaline phosphatase and a diminished urinary calcium excretion. These findings, however, may vary considerably from time to time in the same patient, since the serum calcium and phosphorus levels vary according to the immediate state of vitamin D repletion and small doses can correct the abnormalities rapidly. But the serum alkaline phosphatase follows the bone changes and there is a delay in response to vitamin D. Difficulties in diagnosis also arise in some cases of undoubted osteomalacia because the serum alkaline phosphatase is normal.

Diagnosis

In the majority of cases diagnosis rests on the history of bone pains and muscular weakness, the radiological finding of Looser's zones, typical serum biochemical findings and a history of one of the disorders producing osteomalacia. Radio-stereo assay techniques are now available for measurement of 25-hydroxycholecalciferol levels in the serum, and this estimation should be carried out in doubtful cases. In some patients confirmation of the diagnosis must depend upon histological examination of undecalcified specimens obtained by bone biopsy of the iliac crest.

Treatment

Calciferol should be given orally in doses of 0.025–0.125 mg (1000–5000 i.u.) daily for 1–3 months. In order to counteract the hypocalcaemia occurring immediately after the commencement of treatment (and possibly producing tetany) it is usual to give calcium supplements orally in the form of calcium hydrogen phosphate (1 g) daily. Within 1–2 weeks the serum calcium and inorganic phosphorus reach normal values but the serum alkaline phosphatase does not fall to normal for several months. There is striking symptomatic improvement with disappearance of muscular weakness and bone pains. The Looser's zones gradually heal. When malabsorption is present and it is due to gluten sensitivity a gluten-free diet should be instituted, but the response may be slow over a period of months. If the cause of malabsorption cannot be corrected the oral dose of vitamin D must be much greater, but it is rarely necessary to give it by injection.

OSTEITIS DEFORMANS (PAGET'S DISEASE)

Osteitis deformans, which was described by Sir James Paget in 1877, is a common bone disorder in the elderly affecting 2–4% of people over the age of 60. It is characterized by a combination of excessive bone resorption and deposition. The abnormal processes of bone destruction and overgrowth can result in severe deformity of the skeleton. It can occur at almost any site, but the tibia and the bones of the pelvic girdle and skull are most commonly involved. The polyostotic form of Paget's disease involves multiple areas of the skeleton, but the bone involvement is never generalized. In 10% of cases, Paget's disease is monostotic involving a single bone or a single area.

Clinical features

The affected bones are often enlarged and when long bones are involved they become bowed. Thus characteristic features are enlargement of the skull, and bowing of the tibia, femur and bones of the forearm. Some patients are greatly disabled by severe unremitting bone pain. Transverse fractures, particularly of the shaft of the femur, can occur. Distortion of the bones can lead to pressure on other structures; for example, back pain radiating in a radicular distribution due to pressure on nerve roots, paraplegia due to spinal cord compression (in this case often only one vertebral body is involved) and deafness. In a large number of cases, however, the disease is completely asymptomatic. High output cardiac failure is a rare complication of Paget's disease resulting from multiple small arteriovenous fistulae in areas of affected bone. Cardiac failure is, however, not uncommon in this condition and is usually due to ischaemic heart disease. The most serious complication is the development of osteogenic sarcoma, but this is rare.

Diagnosis

In asymptomatic cases the disease is first revealed by routine X-ray and biochemical screening. The diagnosis is readily made when such features as enlargement of the skull and bowing of long bones are present. Radiographs show cortical thickening, destruction of the normal trabecular pattern and patches of rarefaction and sclerosis. The serum calcium and inorganic phosphorus levels are usually normal, although hypercalcaemia can occur in the active phase of the disease, especially when the patient is immobilized. The serum alkaline phosphatase is characteristically elevated, often markedly so. Urinary hydroxyproline excretion is raised and indicates increased collagen turnover. In men the condition with which Paget's disease is most likely to be confused is sclerotic bone metastases from carcinoma of the prostate.

Treatment

The most effective long-term treatment of Paget's disease is the administration of calcitonin using the porcine, human or salmon hormone. All three hormones have produced a similar degree of clinical, biochemical and radiological improvement, but the salmon and porcine preparations are potentially antigenic. Most patients respond to a dose of 50 MRC units daily given for a period of 3–6 months; thereafter the dosage can usually be reduced to 50 MRC units three times a week. The main indications for treatment are: bone pain; the prevention of hypercalcaemia, hypercalciuria and stone formation due to immobilization; neurological complications with spinal cord compression; high-output cardiac failure, and in the prophylaxis of orthopaedic complications such as protrusia acetabulae in pelvic disease, fracture of the tibia and femur due to lysis in bones, and crippling deformity from the rapid advance of the disease. The effects of treatment in reducing the activity of the disease can be monitored by fall in total hydroxyproline excretion and in the serum alkaline phosphatase levels.

SKELETAL STATUS AND FRACTURES

Fractures in the elderly differ markedly from those in the younger adult, in whom considerable violence, usually direct trauma to the affected part, is required. In the elderly, fractures result from minimal or moderate violence, the site of fracture is usually cancellous bone next to a joint rather than the shaft of a bone, and the incidence is considerably higher in females than in males, especially for fracture of the hip, the lower end of the forearm and of the vertebral bodies.

FEMORAL NECK FRACTURE

Alffram (1964) made an epidemiological analysis of fracture of the hip involving 1664 cases observed over a 13-year period in the population of Malmö. Both in males and females the incidence was negligible below the age of 50, and it apparently doubled for each 5-year increment after the age of 60. The incidence in females was 2.4 times that in males.

Role of osteoporosis

Newton-John and Morgan (1968) were able to show a close parallelism between the fracture rate of the femoral neck and the frequency with which the amount of bone in the population falls below a critical

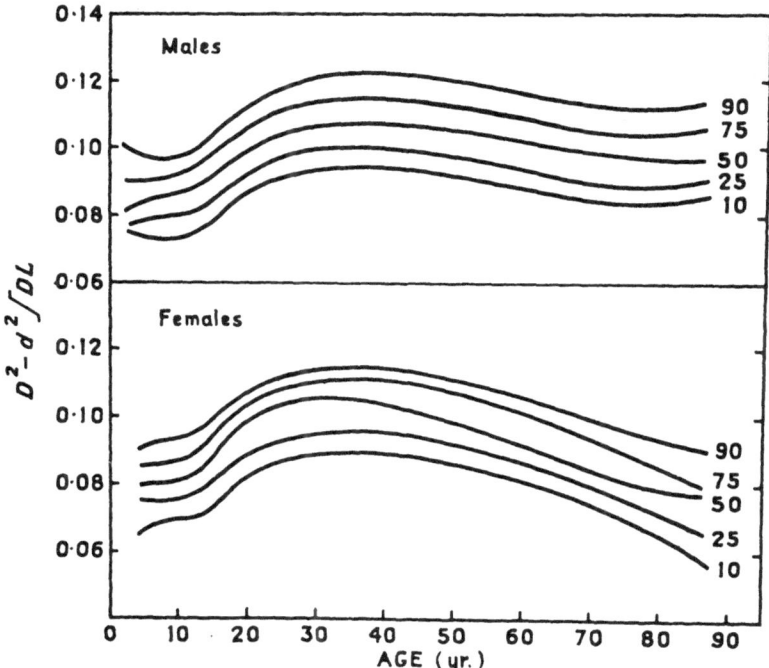

Figure 1 Amount of bone in the second metacarpal; percentile ranking curves for males and females aged 3 to 85 years

283

level. In this and other studies the cortical thickness of the metacarpal was used to estimate the amount of bone. Exton-Smith (1976) calculated the metacarpal cortical ratio based on measurements made on hand radiographs of patients with fracture of the femoral neck. The individual values were plotted on the percentile ranking curves for the general population (see Figure 1). Although the mean values for both the male and female fracture cases were less than those for the general population in the corresponding age groups, and some of the fracture cases had greatly diminished amounts of bone well below the 10th percentiles, there was found to be a wide scatter of values and many were in the higher percentile ranges. These results fail to support the hypothesis that there is a single critical level of bone mass below which fracture of the femoral neck is likely to occur, but there may be a critical level for each individual. The results also indicate that there may be factors other than osteoporosis which contribute to fracture of the femoral neck.

Role of vitamin D deficiency

Aaron *et al.* (1974) in Leeds have shown that 20–30% of women and about 40% of men with fracture of the femoral neck have histological evidence of osteomalacia. Later they showed (Aaron, Gallagher and Nordin, 1974) that the proportion with osteomalacia varied with the season of the year. The highest proportion of bone biopsy specimens with abnormal calcification fronts (43%) was observed in February to April and the lowest (15%) in October to December. The highest frequency of abnormal osteoid-covered surfaces (47%) was observed in April to June and the lowest (13%) in October to December. They conclude that variation in hours of sunshine is responsible for a seasonal change in incidence of femoral neck fractures and possibly for osteomalacia in the elderly population as a whole. The significance of vitamin D deficiency as an important factor in fracture of the proximal femur has been confirmed by the study of Faccini, Exton-Smith and Boyde (1976). The mean value of trabecular osteoid area in the fracture group was 4% compared with 1% in a control group matched for age and sex. The difference was also striking in the portion of trabecular surface covered by osteoid; the mean value for the fracture group was 24.5% compared with 7.9% for the control group. Brown and his colleagues (1976) found significantly lower levels of plasma 25-hydroxycholecalciferol in patients with fracture of the femoral neck compared with those in controls of similar age from whom blood samples were taken at the same time of the year. This is believed to be a reflection of the decreased out-of-doors activity of the patients prior to their fracture.

FRACTURE OF THE WRIST

The effects of age and sex on the incidence of wrist fractures are also clearly seen. There is a high incidence in the young, both in boys and girls, a low incidence in adults and a steep rise in ageing women, unaccompanied by any corresponding change in men. Nordin (1971) compared the radius and ulna 'density' values in normal men and women with the annual age-specific wrist fracture rate in the normal population derived from the data of Knowelden, Buhr and Dunbar (1964). It was found that the fracture rate in the normal population was inversely related to the mean density of the lower end of the radius.

VERTEBRAL COMPRESSION FRACTURES

Measurements of peripheral bone status (for example, in the second metacarpal) in patients with vertebral compression fractures yield inconclusive results. Nevertheless patients with the most severe degrees of osteoporosis of the spine also have low values of bone mass in the metacarpal. Nordin, using spinal densitometry, has shown that crush fracture cases generally suffer from a more severe degree of spinal osteoporosis than other individuals of the same age (Nordin *et al.*, 1968, 1970). He considers that differences between the vertebral and peripheral bone status may depend on the rate at which osteoporosis develops. The vertebral bodies consist largely of trabecular bone, which with its large surface area : volume ratio is preferentially absorbed. Thus in the early stages severe spinal osteoporosis may exist with relatively normal peripheral bones. Peripheral bone loss lags behind the bone resorption in the vertebral bodies.

Thus both osteoporosis and osteomalacia contribute to the rising incidence of fractures in the elderly. In osteomalacia there is an obvious change in the quality of bone, but in osteoporosis there may also be a change in bone quality which is not revealed by histological examination. A complete explanation of the fracture patterns in old age must depend on satisfactory studies of bone-breaking strength and other parameters of bone quality in relation to age and disease states.

II. JOINT DISEASE

AGEING OF JOINTS

Ageing of articular tissues takes place throughout life and the effects become evident after the age of about 25, especially in the weight-bearing joints. Irregularities occur in the surface of the hyaline cartilage which becomes thickened with advancing years. The associated biochemical changes include an increase in the water content, in the quantity of hyaluronic acid and in the ratio of collagen to chondroitin sulphate. By the time old age is reached mucoid degeneration and cyst formation in the matrix are apparent, and calcification of articular cartilage occurs, especially in the knee. The synovial membrane becomes thickened with villous hypertrophy.

OSTEOARTHRITIS

The incidence of osteoarthritis increases markedly with age. In a population survey 87% of females and 83% of males aged between 55 and 64 years showed radiographic evidence of osteoarthritis, but only 22% of the men and 15% of the women had symptoms (Kellgren and Lawrence, 1957).

286

Aetiology

The pathological changes of osteoarthritis are an exaggerated manifestation of the ageing process. It is likely that a vicious circle of cartilage injury is established. The thickened cartilage of older people, mechanically impaired by structural changes, is severely compressed with each normal joint movement. The distortion leads to accelerated breakdown, with the development of fibrillation, cartilage loss, osteophytosis and eburnation of bone.

Clinical features

The onset of symptoms is usually gradual and the condition progresses slowly while the general health of the patient remains good. Contractures and subluxation do not occur and crippling is present, if at all, only in the very advanced stages. In the hands, Heberden's nodes, consisting of hard swellings on the dorsal surface of the terminal phalanges, are the commonest clinical manifestation and are readily recognized. Bouchard's nodes, which are similar lesions over the proximal interphalangeal joints, are often missed.

Generally only one or two joints are sites of symptoms, but many others show typical X-ray changes. The knees, hips and shoulders are affected in this order of frequency; the ankles and wrists are seldom involved. The distribution of pain varies; in the case of the knee it is usually well localized to the joint, but in the case of the hip the pain may be diffuse and referred to the knee or to the buttock and down the back of the thigh so that sciatica is simulated.

Loss of stability in the knee due to disorganization of the joint and laxity of the ligaments may be so marked that the patient complains that his knee 'gives way' while walking. Descent of stairs is often more difficult and painful than is ascent, in which undue movement is prevented by contraction of the muscles. In the later stages, since there is major involvement of the medial compartment, a genu varum deformity may arise and this can produce a serious disturbance of balance. The hypertrophic irregular bones may be palpated and crepitus may be felt on movement. Synovial effusion may occur and lead to the formation of a cystic swelling behind the knee (Baker's cyst). Although the cyst is usually symptomless it can cause local pain and it may compress the popliteal vein.

In osteoarthritis of the hip both sides are affected but impairment of function may be more marked in one hip than in the other. Movement is first limited in abduction and external rotation. The patient with bilateral osteoarthritis of the hip walks with a shuffling gait; there may be difficulty in crossing the legs in sitting; difficulty in rising from a low chair and an inability to bend to tie up shoelaces.

Primary generalized osteoarthritis
Kellgren and Moore (1952) have described a clinical syndrome of generalized osteoarthritis with a distinct pattern of joint involvement. The sites of arthritic change are the distal interphalangeal joints of the fingers, the first carpometacarpal joints, the great toes, the first tarsometatarsal joints, the interfacetal joints of the spine, the knees and hips. Heberden's nodes are a prominent feature. The onset is often acute with tenderness of the joints. The knees in particular may be swollen owing to small effusions. The skin over the joints may be reddened and warm. Pain may be severe and is aggravated by cooling so that patients avoid putting their hands into cold water. In spite of the apparently inflammatory nature of the initial arthritic process there is neither constitutional disturbance nor loss of weight. The erythrocyte sedimentation rate may be moderately raised and this, together with the polyarticular involvement, can lead to a mistaken diagnosis of rheumatoid arthritis. The acute phase subsides in a few months to be followed by a chronic phase characterized by bony outgrowths around the joint margins.

Treatment

Although the articular degenerative changes are irreversible the patient can often be helped by suitable treatment with the relief of symptoms and improvement in joint function. The use of analgesic drugs should be combined with active exercises. There are two main purposes of these active exercises: to improve the range of joint movements and to improve the strength of the muscles responsible for movement of the diseased joints. A wider range of movements, especially at the hip and knee joints, distributes forces over a larger area of articular surface and helps to break the vicious circle which leads to deterioration in the joint condition. In recent years much progress has been made in the surgical treatment of osteoarthritis, and prostheses are available for both hip and knee joint replacement. There is a trend towards arthroplasty and now arthrodesis and osteotomy are less often performed; nevertheless arthrodesis is still required when realignment of the knee is necessary in genu varum.

RHEUMATOID ARTHRITIS

Rheumatoid arthritis not infrequently begins after the age of 60 and, in contrast to the female preponderance of the disease in younger age groups, men are affected almost as often as women. Although radiological changes tend to be more severe in cases of later onset there is usually less deformity and a more benign prognosis.

Clinical features

The onset can be gradual or abrupt and even explosive. Finger joints are often first affected to be followed by involvement of the wrists, ankles, knees, elbows and shoulders. The local symptoms are pain, stiffness, swelling and limitation of movement. Pain is usually severe in the early stages and it is aggravated by movement and ameliorated by rest. Stiffness, which becomes more prominent as the disease progresses, is usually worse in the morning and following periods of rest and it may diminish with exercise. Swelling is due to thickening of the synovial membranes and to small effusions; the bulbous appearance is accentuated by muscular wasting around the joint. The skin over the affected joints may be red and warm but later it becomes thin, shiny and cold.

Geriatrics

The manifestations of the constitutional disturbance which accompanies the disease process include malaise, depression, anorexia, weight loss, mild pyrexia and slowly developing anaemia. Rheumatoid nodules may develop on the elbow joints and on the extensive surface of the forearms. The erythrocyte sedimentation rate is often very high in elderly patients with rheumatoid arthritis and tests for rheumatoid factor often show a high titre, but this is not necessarily associated with a bad prognosis. Another feature of the disease in the older patient is the high incidence of shoulder joint involvement. Indeed, the condition may start with pain and stiffness in the shoulder and hand (simulating the shoulder–hand syndrome); later, however, other joints become involved with the emergence of the typical picture of rheumatoid arthritis. Dislocation of the shoulder may occur in the chronic stages and this is often in an upward direction in the patient who uses a walking frame.

Non-articular manifestations and complications

Other bodily systems besides the joints are involved in rheumatoid disease. The manifestations include pleural effusion, diffuse interstitial pulmonary fibrosis (fibrosing alveolitis), neuropathy, voice changes (due to involvement of the cricoarytenoid joints and to recurrent laryngeal paralysis) and small-vessel arteritis with gangrene of the digits and ulceration, especially of the skin over the dorsal surface of the feet. Anaemia develops and this is resistant to treatment. There is an increased risk of staphylococcal joint infection which may pass unrecognized, especially in patients receiving corticosteroids.

Management

Drugs

Many non-steroidal anti-inflammatory drugs are now available. They have an analgesic effect as well as an anti-inflammatory effect; will reduce joint swelling and the duration of morning stiffness; and will lower the erythrocyte sedimentation rate. Attention must be paid to the total dosage, the time of administration of the drug and the duration of its action. Ideally the patient should have a rapid-acting preparation in the morning with a second dose in the late afternoon, and a long-acting preparation at night in order to ensure sleep and to reduce morning stiffness.

Some of the drugs used in the treatment of rheumatoid arthritis are shown in Table 2. Aspirin has a short duration of action of 4 hours (6–8 hours if enteric coated capsules are used), indomethacin, phenylbutazone and naproxen have a long duration of action of 12 or more hours.

Aspirin has a low therapeutic ratio and often has to be given in a dosage which is near to the toxic level. Monitoring of the blood salicylate level is advisable in the elderly. On the other hand, phenylbutazone has a high therapeutic index and it is often very effective when given in a dose not exceeding 300 mg daily. It can be combined with aspirin. Naproxen also has a high therapeutic ratio and can be given in a twice daily dose. Other non-steroidal anti-inflammatory drugs include ibuprofen, flurbiprofen, indoprofen and sulindac.

Severe rheumatoid disease sometimes responds well to gold. Sodium aurothiomalate (Myocrisin) can be given as 50 mg weekly injection until improvement occurs. The interval between injections for maintenance therapy (50 mg) varies from once a fortnight to once every 3 months. Corticosteroids given orally are now rarely used in the elderly since there is a high incidence of side-effects, especially osteoporotic vertebral collapse in both sexes. Intra-articular injections of hydrocortisone acetate, however, are often very effective when combined with muscle exercises especially in knee and shoulder joint involvement.

General measures

There are probably few other diseases where treatment demands such a careful balance between rest and activity. Prolonged immobilization, especially with faulty positioning, can lead to serious disability and crippling. Nevertheless rest is essential in the active phase with constitutional disturbances. Special attention must be paid to the optimal positioning of affected joints. Light PVC or plastazote splints moulded to the limbs may be required, especially for the wrists and

291

TABLE 2
DRUGS USED IN RHEUMATOID ARTHRITIS

Drug	Usual dose	Adverse effects
Aspirin Enteric coated	8–12 tabs (300 mg)/day 3–14 caps (325 mg) at night	dyspepsia, gastrointestinal haemorrhage, dizziness, tinnitus, skin reactions
Indomethacin	25–50 mg morning 50–100 mg at night	gastrointestinal disturbance, haemorrhage, fluid retention, skin reactions
Phenylbutazone	100 mg twice daily 100 mg at night	gastrointestinal disturbance, haemorrhage, blood dyscrasias, fluid retention, cholestasis
Naproxen	250 mg morning 250–500 mg at night	gastrointestinal disturbance, haemorrhage, fluid retention
Gold Sodium aurothiomalate	50 mg weekly injection (later less frequent injections for maintenance)	renal and hepatic dysfunction, blood dyscrasias, skin rashes and pigmentation
Corticosteroids (a) Oral, e.g. prednisolone	up to 7.5 mg daily	peptic ulceration, haemorrhage, osteoporosis, skin atrophy, predisposition to infection, fluid retention, Cushingoid features
(b) Intra-articular e.g. hydrocortisone	at 6–12-week intervals	articular degeneration simulating neuropathic joint, infection

knees; the weight of the bedclothes on the feet may be reduced by the use of a cradle. The patient is often tempted to place a pillow behind the knees to gain comfort; this must be avoided since slight persistent flexion deformity is the most important single factor in preventing a patient from walking.

As the active phase of the disease passes, a wide variety of exercises should be carried out by the patient. In general these should be related to activities required for daily living. Such active and purposeful exercises are a most valuable means of improving joint function and maintaining muscle strength. Constant encouragement must be given to maintain morale; indeed the patient can be reassured that the crippling disablement which was formerly common can now be avoided by the use of the newer anti-inflammatory drugs.

GOUT

Gout is a disorder of metabolism characterized by recurrent attacks of arthritis and by deposition of sodium urate crystals in soft tissues and bones. Although the first attack of gout usually occurs in middle age, approximately 10% of patients experience their first attack after the age of 60. The chronic deforming changes from gouty arthritis are also seen in older people since the disease is not incompatible with a long life.

Clinical features

The frequency of joint involvement in old age is similar to that occurring in younger patients, namely, the big toe, ankle, fingers, knee, elbow and wrist. The initial sign of this disorder of metabolism is usually an acute attack of gouty arthritis affecting the first metatarsophalangeal joint. The attack is often of great severity, but it eventually subsides completely, leaving the joint in an apparently normal condition. Sometimes several joints are involved simultaneously or in sequence. After a number of episodes the arthritis becomes chronic and deforming with limitation of movement in one or more joints. Deposits of urates in articular structures (synovia, cartilage and tendons) and in the helix of the ear form tophi. The olecranon bursa is a common site to be affected and an irregular painless mass over one elbow in an

293

elderly man should lead to a suspicion of gout. Urate deposits also occur in bones and are seen as small, clean-cut translucent areas on X-ray examination. The usual sites are the head of the metatarsal and the areas immediately adjacent to the phalangeal joints in the hands and feet.

Diagnosis

As is the case in younger patients gout in old age may be precipitated by the use of thiazide diuretics. Some differences in old age are: there is a less frequent positive family history, but gout secondary to blood dyscrasias (usually leukaemia and polycythaemia) is three times more common than in the younger age group; females are affected in about 30% of cases compared with approximately 5% at younger ages; hyperuricaemia (greater than 0.42 mmol/l or 7 mg/100 ml) is usually diagnostic in younger patients but in the elderly elevated serum uric acid levels may be due to renal impairment and to the use of thiazide diuretics.

Treatment

The acute attack may be treated with colchicine, phenylbutazone or indomethacin as in younger patients. Raised plasma uric acid levels associated with repeated attacks of gouty arthritis should be lowered by long-term therapy with uricosuric agents such as probenicid or with the xanthine oxidase inhibitor allopurinol. These drugs are usually well tolerated in old age. In the presence of renal failure or of large tophaceous deposits, and in gout secondary to blood dyscrasia, it is advisable to use allopurinol. With both drugs there is a risk of precipitating an acute attack of gout in the early stages of treatment; this can be minimized by giving small doses (25 mg twice daily) of phenylbutazone concurrently.

PSEUDOGOUT — PYROPHOSPHATE ARTHROPATHY

Although the pathogenetic mechanism is similar, namely an inflammatory reaction provoked by the presence of crystals in the soft tissues, the disease differs from urate gout in a number of ways. It is a disease which becomes increasingly common with advancing years and there is a predilection for involvement of the larger synovial joints, especially the knee. In order to make a diagnosis of pyrophosphate arthropathy a search should be made on radiographic examination for chondrocalcinosis. This is most often seen in the menisci of the knee, the symphysis pubis or in the radio-ulnar joint at the wrist. It appears as a thin line of calcification in the fibrocartilage or synovial membrane. Chondrocalcinosis, however, is common in old age and is not necessarily associated with pyrophosphate arthropathy. There is also a definite association between chondrocalcinosis and the two metabolic disorders, hyperparathyroidism and haemochromatosis; these two disorders must be excluded by appropriate biochemical tests. The diagnosis of pseudo-gout can best be confirmed during the acute attack by examination of synovial fluid aspirate using polarizing microscopy, this will reveal intraleukocytic, positively birefringent crystals of calcium pyrophosphate dihydrate. Treatment of the acute attack consists of the use of phenylbutazone or indomethacin. When the knee joint alone is involved relief can be obtained by aspiration of the synovial effusion.

ARTHROPATHY DUE TO MALIGNANT DISEASE

Myeloproliferative disorders and malignant lymphomas can produce gouty arthritis. The hyperuricaemia is the result of over-production of uric acid due to an increased turnover of nucleoproteins, and it is particularly likely to occur from the use of cytotoxic drugs. When elevated serum uric acid levels are found in these malignant disorders allopurinol should be administered before treatment with cytotoxic agents is started.

In multiple myeloma a polyarthritis of the small joints may occur, and it closely resembles rheumatoid arthritis. The cause is deposition of amyloid in the synovial membrane. When the para-articular tissues are also involved a carpal tunnel syndrome may develop.

Hypertrophic pulmonary osteoarthropathy

This is the most important articular manifestation of malignant disease and in the elderly it is usually due to bronchial carcinoma. The clubbing of the fingers and toes, and the enlargement of the extremities due to periarticular and periosteal thickening, may precede the onset of signs of primary growth. The patient may complain of warmth and burning of the fingertips, painful arthritis, especially of the wrist, and sweating of the hands and feet. X-ray examination of the wrist shows periosteal new bone formation at the lower ends of the radius and ulna. Removal of the tumour may lead to complete resolution; if this is not possible the condition should be treated symptomatically with anti-inflammatory drugs or corticosteroids.

NEUROPATHIC ARTHROPATHY (CHARCOT'S JOINTS)

In diseases of the nervous system associated with impairment or loss of pain sensation destructive lesions of joints can develop. Neuropathic arthropathy should be suspected in elderly patients who have a relatively pain-free joint disease with radiographic changes of joint destruction. New bone formation around the joint is another characteristic X-ray finding in many cases.

The site of the joint involvement varies according to the nature of the neurological disorder. The main causes are:

Tabes dorsalis: with involvement mainly of the hip and knee joints, and occasionally the spine and joints of the upper limb.
Syringomyelia: usually the shoulder and elbow joints are affected.
Diabetic neuropathy: tarsal joints and ankle are mainly affected.
Repeated intra-articular steroid injections: Occasionally in patients who have received repeated intra-articular steroid injections a form of neuropathic arthropathy develops.

The greatest disturbance of joint function occurs when the knee joint is involved. When the hip, spine and feet are the sites of arthropathy the disturbance of function is less apparent, but the radiological findings can be striking.

III. MUSCLE DISORDERS

AGEING IN MUSCLE

The peak of muscle strength occurs between 20 and 30 years, and the decline after maturity shows a progressive acceleration with increasing age. By measurement of hand grip Anderson and Cowan (1966) have defined the relationship between ageing and muscle strength. The predicted power of the grip of the right hand in men decreases from 44.0 kg at the age of 60 years to 32.1 kg at 89 years; the corresponding values at the same ages for women are 32.4 kg and 27.4 kg respectively. The left-hand grip is less than that of the right both in men and women, and the power is greater in men than in women. This decline in muscular strength is regarded as part of physiological ageing, but the rate of decline varies considerably according to the level of physical activity associated with different occupations. Studies of ageing Masai tribesmen (Nilo-Hamitic nomads of Kenya and Tanzania) show that they generally have remarkable muscular strength, often in spite of poor physical health. Without any special training their performances using an electrically driven inclined treadmill have been found to be superior to those of Olympic runners. Decline in muscle strength is usually associated with a parallel decrease in bone density.

MUSCLE WEAKNESS

The complaint of weakness is common in the elderly, especially over the age of 75, but it is difficult to evaluate. Striking weakness is a feature of patients suffering from tuberculosis, renal failure and malignant disease. In congestive cardiac failure and anaemia it is probably due to tissue anoxia. Various metabolic disorders lead to weakness, particularly when associated with hypocalcaemia, hypomagnesiumaemia and hypokalaemia. Muscle weakness and even paralysis can result from a decrease in total body potassium, which in turn may be due to the prolonged uses of thiazide diuretics and purgatives often combined with a low dietary potassium intake.

Sometimes the weakness is most marked in proximal limb and girdle muscles. This form of myopathy is a feature of vitamin D deficiency (see page 278), thyrotoxicosis, Cushing's disease, long-term administration of corticosteroids (cortisone myopathy) and the neuromyopathy of malignant disease, especially carcinoma of the bronchus. Myopathy and muscle-wasting occur in polymyositis and in rheumatoid arthritis.

NOCTURNAL CRAMP

Muscular cramps can occur in people of all ages, but they are more common in the elderly and after the age of 60 some 75% of persons experience cramp. The usual clinical picture is of an individual who retires for the night free from symptoms and is awakened from sleep with severe pain in the calf. The pain is associated with intense contraction of the calf muscles which become hard and tender. The sufferer may gain relief by vigorous rubbing of the affected part or by pressing the foot against the floor. The pain rarely lasts longer than 1 minute, but it may be followed by tenderness in the muscle lasting minutes or even an hour afterwards. Other sites are muscles of the sole of the foot, of the big toe and little toe. The frequency varies greatly in the same individual. When they occur several times in the night or on consecutive nights nocturnal cramps are of importance in disturbing sleep.

The majority of individuals who experience cramp are in a normal state of health. They are more likely to occur in patients suffering from arthritis of the hips or knees, and those who have varicose veins or a history of thrombophlebitis. In those who are predisposed, excessive muscular activity is an important factor favouring the development of cramp. In almost every instance it is noted that exercise taken in excess of the habitual amount during the day is likely to lead to the development of cramp during the rest following this activity (Exton-Smith, 1955).

The essential mechanism is a lasting tetanic contraction of a group of muscle fibres. It may be precipitated by elongation or stretching of the fibres and beyond a certain point the stretch reflex throws the muscle into spasm. Sometimes the muscle stretching may be due to automatic or unconscious movements on awakening from sleep, or to the sudden jerks in the lower limbs which are associated with arthritis of the knees. Such influences, and the fact that they tend to occur during rest following activity, probably account for the nocturnal incidence of muscular cramp.

There are two forms of therapy which have a sound pharmacological basis and are usually effective; these are the use of quinine and mephanesin. Quinine sulphate given in a single dose of 200 mg at bedtime increases the refractory period and diminishes the ability of skeletal muscle to respond to tetanic stimulation. Mephanesin 250–500 mg produces muscle relaxation by diminishing reflex excitability of the spinal cord. Other drugs used in prophylaxis are orphenadrine and diazepam.

POLYMYALGIA RHEUMATICA AND GIANT CELL ARTERITIS

These two disorders are probably different manifestations of the same underlying disease which occur almost entirely in people over the age of 55. Polymyalgia presents with pain and stiffness in the muscles, together with low-grade pyrexia, general malaise and a raised erythrocyte sedimentation rate. The condition may be mistaken for the early stages of rheumatoid arthritis. In giant-cell arteritis similar manifestations are present but the onset is usually with headache, scalp tenderness and palpable inflamed temporal arteries. The clinical picture of this form of arteritis was first described by Jonathan Hutchinson (1890) in the octogenarian father of a London hospital beadle. The patient developed red streaks on the forehead due to inflammation of the temporal arteries. The condition became more widely recognized as a disease entity following the descriptions of a large series of cases by workers at the Mayo Clinic (Horton *et al.*, 1934). Histological examination of affected segments of arteries reveals infiltration of the media with plasma cells, lymphocytes and giant cells together with occlusion of the lumen due to thrombosis or endothelial proliferation. Besides the temporal arteries which are the most frequently involved other arteries affected include: the ophthalmic and retinal arteries responsible for sudden loss of vision; the cerebral arteries producing stroke; the maxillary arteries leading to masticatory angina; and rarely, the nasal arteries causing necrosis of the nasal mucosa. Since the greatest danger is the development of blindness due to ophthalmic arteritis (see page 92) it is important to make a diagnosis with the aim of the earliest possible treatment. The response to steroid therapy is usually dramatic. The initial dosage should be high, e.g. prednisolone 45–60 mg daily, to be followed after a variable time with a maintenance dose sufficient to control symptoms. The disease is self-limiting and after 1–2 years the drug can be withdrawn slowly. If symptoms recur or the ESR rises steroid therapy must be reintroduced.

REFERENCES

Aaron, J E., Gallagher, J. C., Anderson, J., Stasiak, L., Longton, E.B., Nordin, B. E. C. and Nicholson, M. (1974). Frequency of osteomalacia and osteoporosis in fractures of the proximal femur. *Lancet*, **i**, 229

Aaron, J. E., Gallagher, J. C. and Nordin, B. E. C. (1974). Seasonal variation of osteomalacia in femoral neck fractures. *Lancet*, **ii**, 84

Alffram, P. A. (1964). An epidemiological study of cervical and trochanteric fractures of the femur in an urban population. *Acta. Orthop. Scand.* Supp. 65

Anderson, I., Campbell, A. E. R., Dunn, A. and Runciman, J. B. M. (1966). Oseomalacia in elderly women. *Scot. Med. J.*, **11**, 429

Anderson, W. F., and Cowan, N. R. (1966) Handgrip pressure in older people. *Br. J. Prev. Soc. Med.* **20**, 141

Brown, I. R. F., Bakowska, A. and Millard, P. H. (1976). Vitamin D status of patients with femoral neck fractures. *Age and Ageing*, **5**, 127

Chalmers, J., Conacher, W. D. H., Gardner, D. L. and Scott, P. F. (1967). Osteomalacia a common disease in elderly women. *J. Bone Jt. Surg.*, 49B, 403

Davis, M. E., Strandjord, N. M. and Lanzl, L. H. (1966). Estrogens and the aging process. *J. Am. Med. Assoc.*, **196**, 219

Exton-Smith, A. N. (1955). Night cramps in the elderly. *Practitioner*, **175**, 748

Exton-Smith, A. N. (1976). The management of osteoporosis. *Proc. Roy. Soc. Med.*, **69**, 931

Exton-Smith, A. N., Millard, P. H., Payne, P. R. and Wheeler, E. F. (1969). Pattern of development and loss of bone with age. *Lancet*, **ii**, 1154

Faccini, J. M., Exton-Smith, A. N., and Boyde, A. (1976). Disorders of bone and fractures of the femoral neck. *Lancet*, **i**, 1089

Gryfe, C. I., Exton-Smith, A. N., Payne, P. R. and Wheeler, E. F. (1971). Pattern of development of bone in childhood and adolescence. *Lancet*, **i**, 523

Gryfe, C. I., Exton-Smith, A. N. and Stewart, R. J. C. (1972). Determination of the amount of bone in the metacarpal. *Age and Ageing*, **1**, 213

Horton, B. T., Magath, T. B. and Brown, G. E. (1934). Arteritis of the temporal vessels. *Arch. Intern. Med.*, **53**, 400

Hutchinson, J. (1890). Diseases of the arteries. *Arch. Surg. Lond.*, **1**, 323

Jowsey, J., Riggs, B. L., Kelly, P. J. and Hoffman, D. L. (1972). Effect of combined therapy with sodium fluoride, vitamin D and calcium in osteoporosis. *Am. J. Med.*, **53**, 43

Kellgren, J. H. and Lawrence, J. S. (1957). Radiological assessment of osteoarthrosis. *Ann. Rheum. Dis.*, **16**, 494

Kellgren, J. H. and Moore, R. (1952). Primary generalised osteoarthrosis. *Br. Med. J.*, **1**, 181

Knowelden, J., Buhr, A. J. and Dunbar, O. (1964). Incidence of fractures in persons over 35 years of age. *Br. J. Prev. Soc. Med.*, **18**, 130

Newton-John, H. F. and Morgan, D. B. (1968). Osteoporosis: disease or senescence? *Lancet*, **i**, 232

Nordin, B. E. C. (1971). Clinical significance and pathogenesis of osteoporosis. *Br. Med. J.*, **1**, 571

Nordin, B. E. C., Young, M. M., Bentley, B., Oromondroyd, P. and Sykes, J. (1968). Lumbar spine densitometry. *Clin. Radiol.*, **19**, 459

Nordin, B. E. C., Young, M. M., Bulusu, L. and Horsman, A. (1970). In U. S. Barzel (ed). *Osteoporosis*. (New York: Grune and Stratton)

Paget, J. (1877). On a form of chronic inflammation of bones (osteitis deformans), *Med. Chir. Trans.*, **60**, 37

15
Rehabilitation with special reference to stroke

Rehabilitation of the stroke patient is a neglected subject in most medical schools. All too often the patient is regarded as an embarrassment for whom the doctor can do nothing, and the field is left open to the various remedial therapists to do the best they can. This is a sad state of affairs, since even if hard scientific evidence showing an advantage to the patient treated by a team skilled in stroke rehabilitation is hard to come by, there is little doubt that the enthusiasm and morale of such teams tend to be high. Many stroke patients have benefited from the work of teams skilled in rehabilitation.

There is a high mortality in the first 3 weeks following a stroke: anywhere between one-third and one-half of patients die. The prognosis for life of the survivors is good, but approximately half will have a residual defect and will require some help with walking or daily living activities, a quarter will need constant nursing care and a long-stay hospital bed, and only a quarter will make a total recovery. Thus there is an ever-growing pool of disabled stroke survivors in the community and increasing pressure on hospital resources. It has been estimated that between 1973 and 1991 the number of bed-days occupied by patients with cerebrovascular disease will rise from 11.2% of the annual total to 17.3% an increase of 65% (Garraway and Akthar, 1978).

It must be stressed that the various disciplines involved with a stroke patient cannot work in isolation. A coordinated, planned approach avoids waste of time and effort, avoids misunderstanding and allows everyone to see his own role in relation to others. It is convenient here to look at the individuals involved to see what special responsibilities each has within the team.

DOCTOR

The doctor must ensure that the patient has been fully assessed and that any 'hidden disabilities' which may delay rehabilitation are fully explained to the rest of the team. Thus a patient who is labelled as 'difficult and lazy' may have serious impairment of concentration and short-term memory to account for his apparent refusal to respond.

Mental barriers

Dementia is the profoundest of these barriers. Although tests of mental function can be difficult or impossible to use in aphasic patients some attempt must be made to assess orientation and the level of comprehension. Isaacs and Marks (1973) have described three tests, which when performed badly indicate a significantly poorer chance of the patient recovering sufficiently to leave hospital. These are:

(1) *The set test*: the patient is asked to tell the examiner all the colours he can think of. One point is scored for each correct answer to a maximum of 10. Similarly for animals, fruits and towns, making a maximum of 40.
(2) *Three blocks*: the patient is given toy building blocks of diminishing size and told to build the blocks, one on top of the other, to form a column. If the patient fails the examiner demonstrates and then invites him to try again.
(3) *Posting box*: the toy posting box has six holes cut in the lid with

six corresponding shapes to be posted through. Not only is this a test of comprehension but by positioning the box in different halves of the patient's visual field it can be used as a test of visual neglect.

Short-term memory can be assessed by asking the patient to repeat what the examiner has just asked him to do. Clearly if it is poor the patient is severely handicapped in following instructions from a nurse or physiotherapist. Depression is a common consequence of a stroke and must be looked for. It should be differentiated from four other behavioural changes associated with cerebrovascular disease: emotional lability, a general loss of confidence, a determination to give up and do no more and emotional incontinence where there are outbursts of weeping or laughter unrelated to the underlying affect (Hurwitz and Adams, 1972).

Sensory defects

The patient's hearing and visual acuity should be checked (have his hearing aid or spectacles been lost or forgotten?) as well as evidence of hemianaesthesia or proprioceptive loss. Hemianopia is rarely a major problem since the patient will compensate by moving his head or eyes. Visual neglect is more serious as the patient is unaware of the defect. It may be tested for by using two pens of different colours which are held about 10 inches apart and 10 inches in front of the patient, who is asked what he sees. The two pens are then interchanged and the question repeated. Patients with visual neglect report seeing only the pen on the unaffected side, whilst the hemianopic patient will shift his field of vision in order to view both pens (Isaacs and Marks, 1973).

Sensory neglect, like visual neglect, is nearly always a result of a non-dominant hemisphere lesion and thus affects the left side of the body. It will be found that, although touch is felt on the affected side when there is a single stimulus, it will not be experienced when both sides of the body are touched simultaneously.

Disturbances of body image

This is a serious handicap to the successful rehabilitation of the stroke patient. It is caused by a lesion to the non-dominant parietal lobe and is thus most frequently seen in patients with a left hemiparesis. The presence of this disability, together with the other effects of non-dominant parietal lobe lesions such as sensory neglect and constructional apraxia, explains why a patient with a left hemiparesis is often more difficult to rehabilitate than one with a right hemiparesis. It may be tested for by asking the patient to draw a man, a house or a clock. The drawing of a man may reveal gross defects in the positioning of the limbs and if sensory neglect is also present it is usual for the left side of the drawing to be omitted.

Apraxia

This is a loss of ability to initiate purposive movements at will even in limbs that are not paralysed, or to perform a previously learned skilled act, although comprehension, motor power, coordination and sensation are intact (Adams and Hurwitz, 1963). Constructional apraxia is a feature of a non-dominant parietal lobe lesion and is revealed as a difficulty in the patient's ability to dress. He gets into a muddle with buttons and which arm to put into which sleeve of his shirt or jacket. It may be tested for by asking the patient to copy simple designs made of matches (e.g. triangles and squares).

Lesions of the dominant parietal lobe tend to produce a bilateral apraxia, in particular effecting movements of the lips and tongue. Petren's gait, an apraxic gait, may be seen, where the patient has great difficulty in initiating walking. By coaxing he may be persuaded to take a few small-paced steps, but interestingly a longer stride may often be achieved by asking the patient to step across lines drawn on the floor at 18-inch intervals.

NURSE

Because nurses are with the patient all the time they are in a very

306

strong position to assist rehabilitation by ensuring correct positioning and to prevent bad habits developing during sitting or transferring. From the earliest stages abnormal postures must be corrected to prevent increased spasticity, contractures and pressure sores. Thus, typical postures which should be prevented include: side flexion of the trunk on the affected side, head flexion to the affected side, depression of the shoulder, flexion and pronation of the forearms and flexion at wrist and fingers and either flexion and adduction, or extension and adduction, of the leg.

The bedside locker, food, visitors and nursing procedures should be on the patient's affected side (although in the early stages with a patient who has visual and sensory neglect this approach may have to be modified).

When sitting the patient in a chair it is important to ensure that he is sitting well back, with his head and trunk upright, weight evenly distributed and the affected arm supported forwards on a pillow. Learning the correct position for transfers in bed not only reduces the number of nurses who report sick with back strain but ensures the patient's safety and confidence.

Care with the affected shoulder is important to prevent painful shoulder–hand syndrome. The patient should never be pulled by his affected arm nor should it be supported in a sling. A sling does not prevent subluxation and only reinforces the spastic pattern of flexion. Instead the patient should be encouraged to interlace his fingers with palms together and elbows extended, and frequently lift both arms up above his head.

In addition to these activities the nurse does, of course, have her more traditional and equally important role: care of skin and pressure areas (see Chapter 15) and ensuring adequate hydration. Some patients are only incontinent because they are unable to ask for a urinal or bedpan and the skilled nurse will avoid these humiliating episodes for the patient by regularly offering the appropriate receptacle. Enemas or a suppository may be necessary to open the bowels.

Above all the nurse encourages the patient to have a positive, independent outlook. It is very time-consuming to stand and allow the patient to do things for himself but it is the best way towards functional recovery. Relatives and friends have to be instructed on this point. For instance it is better to tell them not to feed the patient but to allow him to do it himself even if it takes an hour and most of the food ends up on the floor. The relatives should be given the definite expectation that the patient will return home and be encouraged to help and learn from the nurses on the ward. Although at first many relatives find the prospect of caring for a stroke patient at home as too daunting a responsibility, nurses have had some remarkable successes after weeks of patient teaching and demonstration on the ward.

PHYSIOTHERAPIST

The physiotherapist should probably spend as much time teaching the nursing staff and others the correct procedures for positioning and lifting as on directly working with the patient. Bad habits once developed by the patients can take a long time to correct.

Broadly speaking the aims of physiotherapy are: to establish correct positioning, inhibit spasticity, prevent deformity, restore a normal pattern of movement, increase strength and endurance, improve coordination and balance and to assist the patient towards a high quality of life rather than mere functional independence.

The physiotherapist is concerned with preventing muscle spasm whilst balance and coordination are re-established. On the affected side the normal postural reflex mechanism is absent so that righting reactions, equilibrium reactions and muscle tone are all affected. These reflex mechanisms are not present at birth but develop during infancy, and similarly the hemiplegic patient, through rolling, crawling, kneeling and standing, re-learns postural control and the ability to initiate movement from the affected side (Johnstone, 1976).

Various approaches have been developed by physiotherapists. Bobarth (1970) stresses the importance of inhibiting abnormal reflexes so as to allow normal patterns of movement to emerge. By adopting certain positions it is possible to reduce abnormal reflexes as well as spasticity generally. The technique of proprioceptive neuro-muscular facilitation (PNF) (Knott and Voss, 1968) is a method of promoting the response of the neuromuscular mechanism through stimulation of the proprioceptors. The exercises that are most effective are those which permit maximum elongation of related muscle groups so that the stretch reflex is elicited. These exercises are spiral and diagonal and are related to normal functional movements.

The physiotherapist will employ various aids. A quadruped walking aid (a stick with four feet) may be needed if the patient has not developed full standing balance. The disadvantage of the aid is that the patient leans on it and circumducts the affected leg whilst the affected arm is drawn up in flexor spasm. This can be prevented by the physiotherapist walking on the patient's affected side, holding his arm whilst getting him to lean towards her so that the affected leg bears weight. Pressure splints may be needed to re-establish proprioceptive sensation. Short leg braces are sometimes needed if the leg is flaccid or if the toe drags, but should not be used routinely.

OCCUPATIONAL THERAPIST

The main function of the occupational therapist is to re-educate the patient in the normal activities of daily living (ADL). She is skilled in correcting, or helping the patient to adjust to perceptual problems, and coordinates with the physiotherapist in improving balance and the functional range of movements of the limbs. She will also assess the patient for a wheelchair, if necessary, and train him in its use. Most importantly she will visit the patient's home and advise on any aids or alterations that will be needed.

Dressing is only one of the many activities of daily living, but it is a good example of an area in which relatives can be encouraged to play a part. This should initially be done on the ward under supervision, the aim being that the relative gains sufficient confidence to be able to cope when the patient is at home. The following notes are designed for the relative of a stroke patient and have been prepared by Miss C.

Geriatrics

Hough, Head Occupational Therapist at St Pancras Hospital.

(1) Allow plenty of time in an area where you will be undisturbed.
(2) Choose simple clothes in lightweight and stretch fabrics that have easy fastenings. Adaptations to buttons using Velcro or to cuffs using two buttons joined by elastic thread, ties made up and stitched to elastic.
(3) Place clothing where the patient can see it. Later, if there is a partial loss of vision, you may try to help the patient to learn to compensate for this by moving the clothing slightly out of his range of vision and getting him to turn his head.
(4) Start dressing on the bed and progress to sitting on the side of the bed or in a chair. Be sure that the patient has plenty of support.
(5) Put the affected arm/leg into the sleeve/pants first, so that the unaffected limb is free to assist.
(6) Use braces to pull up trousers or put loops on to underwear.
(7) Shoes, stockings and socks can be put on by lifting the affected foot across the other or on to a footstool. This is often the most difficult stage in dressing.
(8) Slip-on shoes may be preferred but whatever the choice ensure that they give good support to the foot. Elastic shoelaces may be bought or the one-handed method learnt.
(9) A full length mirror gives the patient the opportunity to observe mistakes and to notice his improvements.
(10) Have the patient aim to dress so that he feels satisfied with his appearance.

SPEECH THERAPIST

The problems facing a stroke patient who discovers that he is aphasic have been likened to being hit on the head and waking up in a strange place where everyone is speaking a strange language and where you cannot make yourself understood. If, in addition, everyone insists on treating you as an imbecile it is not surprising if you become anxious,

310

frightened and frustrated.

In addition to determining the exact nature of the patient's speech disturbance and working directly with him to help overcome it, the speech therapist has the important task of explaining to relatives, and the rest of the rehabilitation team, the nature of the disability and how everyone who comes in contact with the patient can help.

Different patients have different problems and one must never forget to treat the patient and not the disability. Some patients have dysarthria, others a receptive or expressive dysphasia. There may be problems in reading and it can be difficult for the person even to write his name. A few general guidelines are:

(1) An encouraging, positive approach is best, but avoid artificial praise.

(2) Keep your own speech slow and simple but never childish. Unless the patient was deaf before his stroke there is no need to raise your voice.

(3) Encourage the patient to talk and give him plenty of time to respond. Do not keep on putting words into his mouth.

(4) Aphasia as such does not alter the patient's basic intelligence, and if speech is difficult try showing him objects and pictures and encourage him to point to the things he wants.

(5) Let him know when his attempts at speech are successful and encourage him to continue. Minimize correction and criticism.

(6) If you are relaxed and unhurried this will in turn reduce the patient's apprehensions and tension.

(7) Keep background noise to a minimum (e.g. television and radio) and watch out for minor distractions that pass unnoticed by you but preoccupy the patient (Porch, 1976).

There have been encouraging results with the use of volunteers in the treatment of aphasia. The speech therapist diagnoses, assesses and guides treatment, but anyone who is willing to talk to and listen to the patient regularly can be of great practical help.

SOCIAL WORKER

The family member who suffers a stroke loses his accustomed role within the family circle. The remaining members are shocked, bewildered and anxious, and react in different ways to this new situation. There may be guilt because a relative has handed over the responsibility for care to the hospital and this can be expressed as unreasonable criticisms of the nursing staff. Dormant problems within the family may be highlighted by this illness. One relative may feel that she is having to carry too much of the responsibility for visiting, another may think the patient has gone 'senile' and becomes angry, frustrated or over-anxious.

The social worker must spend a considerable amount of time in counselling and helping the patient's relatives. She also has to support the patient and discuss, at the appropriate time, plans for discharge. This may be to home where there will be a need to organize community services: home helps, meals-on-wheels, day centres, etc; or it may be to a residential or nursing home. Successful placing of an old person in a residential home calls for a great deal of skill and care. It is not merely a question of filling in a form. The patient must understand and accept the move and may need, on several occasions, to have the chance to express his fears and doubts. The patient should be matched (ideally) with a home in the right neighbourhood, where there is a suitable mix of residents and where he and the staff have compatible temperaments. Once in the home he will need help to adjust and settle in. It must be stressed that a social worker should be asked to visit the stroke patient during his first week of admission and not 6 months later when it is time for 'disposal'. Then there is time for her to develop a rapport with patient and relatives and be in a good position to help and advise.

VOLUNTEER

An enthusiastic voluntary help organizer and his team can make an enormous difference to the stroke patient's life. Outings to the seaside,

312

farm, theatre or brewery remind the patient of life outside hospital and get him away for a while from 'the symbol of sickness' – his bed. On the ward there are cats, budgerigars and fish that can be contemplated, fed and groomed. A bird table outside the window with bird charts to help with identification, growing tomatoes or flowers in window boxes and the whole world of painting, pottery and modelling can be offered the patient with voluntary help.

REFERENCES

Adams, G. F. and Hurwitz, L. J. (1963). Mental barriers to recovery from stroke. *Lancet*, **ii**, 533

Bobarth, B. (1970). *Adult Hemiplegia: Evaluation and Treatment.* (London: Heinemann)

Garraway, M. and Akthar, A. J. (1978). Theory and practice of stroke rehabilitation In B. Isaacs (ed.). *Recent Advances in Geriatric Medicine.* (Edinburgh: Churchill Livingstone)

Hurwitz, L. J. and Adams, G. F. (1972). Rehabilitation of hemiplegia: indices of assessment and prognosis. *Br. Med. J.*, **1**, 94

Isaacs, B. and Marks, R. (1973). Determinants of outcome of stroke rehabilitation. *Age and Ageing*, **2**, 139

Johnstone, M. (1976). *The Stroke Patient: Principles of Rehabilitation.* (Edinburgh: Churchill Livingstone)

Knott, M. and Voss, D. E. (1968). *Proprioceptive Neuromuscular Facilitation: Patterns and Techniques.* 2nd edn. (New York: Harper and Row)

Porch, B. E. (1976). Communication. In G. G. Hirschberg, L. Lewis and P. Vaughan (eds.). *Rehabilitation.* 2nd edn. (Philadelphia: Lippincott)

313

16
Principles of drug therapy

Early pioneers in geriatrics showed what could be achieved in the management of seemingly 'hopeless' cases. Principles of rehabilitation of hemiplegia and other locomotor disorders were evolved, and the ill-effects of immobilization of the elderly in bed were recognized and avoided. More recently, a major contribution of the specialty to medicine as a whole has been a fuller understanding of the possibilities of treatment of elderly patients, and many old people have benefited from a more optimistic and active therapeutic endeavour. A more thorough investigation of patients reveals the silent existence of many conditions and that multiple pathology is the rule rather than the exception. Treatment of these multiple disorders has, however, led to new problems resulting from the administration to the individual patient of a number of powerful drugs which may produce a variety of ill effects.

THERAPEUTIC HAZARDS

A survey conducted in hospitals in Belfast disclosed an incidence of drug reactions of 10.2% in the 1160 patients who were receiving drug therapy (Hurwitz and Wade, 1969). The incidence of reactions was 15.4% in those over the age of 60 compared with 6.3% in those under this age. Hurwitz (1969) also found that 2.9% of patients were admitted to hospital because of adverse reactions to drugs, and the median age of these patients was 60 years.

It is not surprising, therefore, that the admission of many elderly patients is precipitated by inappropriate drug treatment and complications of treatment often arise during the course of the patients' stay in hospital. Such problems arise particularly in elderly patients being treated for congestive cardiac failure, diabetes mellitus, arthritis and mental disturbances. The variety of therapeutic hazards in the elderly, and the factors responsible for them, deserve special emphasis.

Almost all drugs have multiple actions; once absorbed into the body some action is exerted on all cells. The 'specific' action of the drug is the desired action occurring at a tissue concentration of the drug before other actions begin. Fortunately, in most circumstances the safety margin is wide and the untoward actions do not occur. The degree to which tissues tolerate the action of drugs depends on the intactness of cells, and reduced tolerance to drugs may be due to senescence, disease or both. So-called toxic reactions (excluding idiosyncrasy) are in reality the total action of the drug, and in old age the undesired reactions appear more often and sooner.

THE PHYSICIAN'S ROLE IN GOOD THERAPEUTICS

The physician's responsibility for the proper treatment of elderly patients can be considered under two headings (Table 1). He must have a good knowledge of the effects of senescence and of disease on the pharmacokinetics of drugs, and he must evaluate in the individual patient the many factors which may alter his response to drugs.

I. EFFECTS OF SENESCENCE AND DISEASE

1. Drug absorption and transport

The precise extent to which the absorption of drugs from the gastrointestinal tract is affected by changes in gastrointestinal function in old

316

TABLE 1

PRINCIPLES OF DRUG TREATMENT

I. Effects of senescence and disease
 1. Drug absorption and transport
 2. Drug metabolism
 3. Drug excretion
 4. Target organ sensitivity

II. The physician's evaluation
 1. Accurate diagnosis
 2. Possibilities of drug interactions
 3. Indirect effect of drugs
 4. Avoidance of over-medication
 5. Supervision of long-term medication

age is unknown (Bender, 1968). Any reduction in absorption is usually accompanied by decreased metabolism and excretion. Thus limited absorption from the intestine is balanced by delayed elimination of drugs.

The age-related decline in serum albumin concentration produces significant increases in the free levels of drugs which are strongly bound to protein, for example salicylates, sulphadiazine and phenylbutazone. Side-effects of steroid therapy are frequent in patients with low serum albumin levels.

2. Drug metabolism

The microsomal enzyme system in the liver is the primary site of drug metabolism. The duration of action of drugs is determined by the rate at which they are metabolized. The drug which has been most extensively studied in the elderly is antipyrine. Its rapid absorption, distribution, low protein-binding and its elimination almost entirely by metabolism in the liver make it useful for studies of hepatic drug

317

metabolism. In many elderly people the rates of metabolism of anti-pyrine, and to a lesser extent of paracetamol and phenylbutazone, are greatly reduced. O'Malley and his colleagues (1971) have shown that the mean plasma half-life of antipyrine and phenylbutazone is 45% and 20% greater respectively in the elderly compared with that in younger controls. Briant and co-workers (1976) showed that although the mean half-life of paracetamol was significantly longer in the old than in the young (2.2 hours and 1.78 hours respectively) there was considerable overlap in the individual values for the two age groups. Thus individual variability may be as important as differences due to age.

3. Drug excretion

For many drugs (for example, most antibiotics and cardiac glycosides) the kidney may be virtually the sole route of elimination, and for others renal excretion may deal with a significant fraction. Impairment of renal function associated with ageing (see Chapter 10) will have important pharmacokinetic implications for many therapeutic agents. Apart from this physiological decline many elderly patients show an additional decrement in renal function due to dehydration, congestive cardiac failure and renal disease. For drugs with a high therapeutic ratio changes in renal function are of relatively little importance, but for drugs such as digoxin with a low therapeutic ratio the dosage in the elderly must be considerably reduced.

The plasma half-life of digoxin is lengthened by 40% in elderly people compared with the young (Ewy *et al.*, 1969). Taylor and his colleagues (1974) measured serum digoxin concentrations in seven elderly patients during digitalization with digoxin 0.25 mg daily, without a loading dose. Serum concentrations in the therapeutic range (1–2 ng/ml) were reached in 4 days in five patients with normal renal function, while 'toxic' levels (of 3 ng/ml and above) were reached in the same time in two patients with renal impairment.

4. Target organ sensitivity

An increased drug effect is sometimes due to a greater sensitivity of the receptor sites in old people. Castleden and his colleagues (1977) have shown by means of psychometric tests an increased sensitivity of the ageing brain to 10 mg nitrazepam despite similar plasma levels and half-lives of the drug in old and young subjects. Phenothiazines are believed to inhibit noradrenergic and dopaminergic receptor sites in the central and autonomic nervous system, and the liability to side-effects (Parkinsonism and postural hypotension) from the use of phenothiazines appears to be greater in older patients compared with the young. It is believed that physiological decline in autonomic function, which is known to increase in frequency with advancing age, commonly interacts with other factors such as the use of potentially hypotensive drugs to produce postural hypotension in old age. An age-related decline in autonomic function also accounts for the greater liability of the elderly to develop hypothermia under conditions of cold stress, and this impairment of temperature homeostasis is responsible for the greater susceptibility of the elderly to the hypothermic effects of phenothiazine tranquillizers (Exton-Smith, 1973). The potential danger of phenothiazines in inducing heat illness in old people has recently been described (Ellis, 1976).

It is well known that potassium depletion causes increased sensitivity of the heart to digoxin. It commonly occurs following the use of powerful diuretics in the treatment of cardiac failure, but a supplementary factor in some old people is a reduced intake due to a poor diet. The serum potassium is only a rough guide to the total body potassium, but low serum levels are nearly always associated with low total body levels.

II. THE PHYSICIAN'S EVALUATION

1. Accurate diagnosis

An incorrect diagnosis is made in many elderly patients with congestive cardiac failure, left ventricular failure, pneumonia and urinary tract infections, especially when mental symptoms are the presenting feature. Such patients may be given inappropriate psychotropic medication with consequent worsening of their mental and physical state. Mild, and even severe, degrees of mental impairment are often missed in the elderly, and it is good practice to carry out serial mental test scores as a routine in the overall assessment of the older patient.

2. *Possibility of drug interactions*

Interaction between drugs is a relatively uncommon problem in the younger patient suffering from a single disease. In the elderly patient with multiple pathological processess simultaneous treatment with more than one drug is often required. Drug interactions may occur at a number of sites:

(a) *Delayed absorption*
Tricyclic antidepressants which have anticholinergic properties decrease gastrointestinal motility and interfere with the absorption of other drugs.

(b) *Competitive protein-binding*
Phenylbutazone and salicylates probably enhance the hypoprothrombinaemic effects of warfarin by displacing it from the protein-binding site, and highly protein-bound drugs such as sulphonamides and oxyphenbutazone have the potential to displace a moderately protein-bound drug such as tolbutamide enhancing its effect.

(c) *Altered metabolism*
Barbiturates and anticonvulsant drugs (especially sodium diphenylhydantoin) cause hepatic enzyme induction which may interfere with the hydroxylation of vitamin D with the production of osteomalacia.

(d) *Interaction at receptor sites*
Phenothiazines and antihistamines have atropine-like effects and may prevent acetylcholine reaching its receptor sites, thus causing symptoms of urinary retention, blurred vision and ileus; these symptoms are especially common in patients with prostatic enlargement, glaucoma and constipation.

320

3. Indirect effects of drugs

Adverse effects can arise as secondary consequences of the actions of a drug. These mechanisms are of special importance in the elderly since such effects consist of the precipitation of latent disease which is often more prevalent and more often undetected in the elderly patient. Common examples are: the unmasking of diabetes by steroids and thiazide diuretics, the precipitation of acute gout by thiazides, the reactivation of chronic tuberculosis by steroid therapy, the induction of hypothyroidism by iodides, phenylbutazone and para-aminosalicylic acid, and the precipitation of myocardial infarction by thyroxine in the treatment of myxoedema.

4. Avoidance of over-medication

For reasons which have already been discussed there is a greater individual variation in response to drugs in old age compared with that seen in younger patients. Thus the threshold for side-effects is often lowered in the elderly, and the dose regime required to produce a therapeutic effect may also be lowered. In youth the 'normal' response to therapeutic doses of a drug is comparatively well-defined and apart from idiosyncrasies the majority of individuals will show this response. In old age, however, the response is likely to vary from the hypothetical normal.

Indeed for many drugs each prescription given to an older patient should be regarded as an individual therapeutic experiment. Digitalis toxicity is one of the commonest adverse reactions encountered in the elderly; for the older patient an effective maintenance dose of digoxin can be as small as 0.0625 mg per day. According to Dall (1970) maintenance digoxin therapy is probably unnecessary in about 70% of cases.

5. Supervision of long-term medication

Many elderly patients receive unnecessary maintenance doses of drugs; for example, a survey in a psychiatric hospital has shown that about 80% of elderly patients with dementia continue to receive tranquillizers unnecessarily (Barton and Hurst, 1968). Repeat prescriptions are often given to elderly patients suffering from chronic diseases without adequate surveillance of the drug regimen and adequate assessment of changes in clinical state. Elderly patients with such illnesses as hypertension and diabetes mellitus which have been acquired at a younger age may receive year after year the same therapeutic regime, yet it is known that the insulin requirement of diabetics often falls in old age and hypertension after the age of 70 has no effect on longevity (Hodkinson and Exton-Smith, 1976). Not only may vigorous antihypertensive therapy produce severe side-effects in the elderly, but the reduction in cerebral blood flow in the presence of cerebral arterial disease may aggravate ischaemia of the brain.

CORRECT PRESCRIBING

Adherence to several principles is essential if therapeutic hazards are to be avoided and optimum benefit is to be obtained from drug treatment in the elderly:

(1) A full assessment of the elderly patient is essential. This should include evaluation of renal function, especially when drugs prescribed for the patient are those for which the main route of excretion is the kidney. In some cases, particularly for patients receiving psychotropic drugs, it is desirable to withdraw current therapy to ascertain whether improvement in physical and mental condition will occur.

(2) The physician should have a basic knowledge of the pharmacokinetics of the drugs he is prescribing. When the half-life of a drug is likely to be prolonged and the serum levels elevated by reduction in the rate of metabolism in the liver or of the excretion by the kidneys, the dosage must generally be much lower than that usually given to a younger patient. This is particularly important for drugs with a low therapeutic ratio such as digoxin.

(3) Therapeutic regimes should be as simple as possible, both in the number of drugs prescribed and in the frequency of administration. In some cases, however, it is advantageous to give a combination of drugs since it allows a satisfactory response to be obtained with a smaller dose of the more potent therapeutic agent; for example, the combination of a hypotensive agent with a thiazide diuretic.

(4) Repeat prescriptions should only be given after careful reassessment of the patient's clinical state.

(5) Errors in self-medication by elderly patients at home can be reduced by the use of a tear-off calendar and/or a tablet identification card as a memory aid (Wandless and Davie, 1977) or by the use of a drug dispenser (Keet, 1976). Even with these aids, many confused elderly patients will require careful supervision by relatives, neighbours or community nurses.

REFERENCES

Barton, R., and Hurst, L. (1968). Unnecessary use of tranquillizers in elderly patients. *Br. J. Psychiat.*, **112**, 989

Bender, A. D. (1968). Effect of age on intestinal absorption: implications for drug absorption in the elderly. *J. Am. Geriatr. Soc.*, **16**, 1331

Briant, R. H., Dorrington, R. E., Cleal, J. and Williams, F. (1976). The rate of acetaminophen metabolism in the elderly and the young. *J. Am. Geriatr. Soc.*, **24**, 359

Castleden, C. M., George, C. F., Marcer, D., and Hallet, C. (1977). Increased sensitivity to nitrazepam in old age. *Br. Med. J.*, **1**, 10

Dall, J. L. (1970). Maintenance digoxin in the elderly. *Br. Med. J.*, **2**, 705

Ellis, F. (1976). Heat wave deaths and drugs affecting temperature regulation. *Br. Med. J.*, **3**, 474

Exton-Smith, A. N. (1973) Accidental hypothermia, *Br. Med. J.*, **4**, 727

Ewy, G. A., Kapadia, G. G., Yao, L., Lullin, M. and Marcus, F. I. (1969). Digoxin metabolism in the elderly. *Circulation*, **39**, 449

Hodkinson, H. M. and Exton-Smith, A. N. (1976). Factors predicting mortality in the elderly in the community. *Age and Ageing*, **5**, 110

Hurwitz, N. (1969). Admissions to hospital due to drugs, *Br. Med. J.*, **1,** 539

Hurwitz, N. and Wade, O. L. (1969). Intensive hospital monitoring of adverse reactions to drugs. *Br. Med. J.*, **1,** 531

Keet, J. (1976) Failure of the elderly to take medications as prescribed and ways to improve compliance. *Medical Annual*. (Bristol: John Wright)

O'Malley, K., Crooks, J., Duke, E. and Stevenson, I. H. (1971). Effect of age and sex on human drug metabolism. *Br. Med. J.*, **3,** 607

Taylor, B. B., Kennedy, R. D. and Caird, F. I. (1974). Digoxin studies in the elderly. *Age and Ageing*, **3,** 79

Wandless, I. and Davie, J. W. (1977). Can drug compliance in the elderly be improved? *Br. Med. J.* **1,** 359

17
Care of the dying patient

There has recently been a renewed interest shown by the medical and lay press in the manner in which a person dies. Much of this interest reflects an awareness that sociological changes have produced an atmosphere in which death is a taboo subject. These changes are many and complex: the decline of formalized religion, the unrealistic expectations encouraged by a consumer-orientated society, and the growth of a complex health care system in which, with each new 'breakthrough', there is the promise of eventual victory over death. One of the results is that more and more people are dying, not at home among relatives and friends, but in a hospital amid the paraphernalia of last-ditch resuscitation attempts. Thus Ivan Illich (1975) can write: 'The medicalisation of society has brought the epoch of natural death to an end. Western man has lost the right to preside at his act of dying'.

However, this is not to argue that doctors should stand idly by the terminally-ill patient; rather it is to emphasize that, even when treatment to prolong life has been abandoned as inappropriate, the dying patient is still in need of skilled, compassionate care.

The processes which patients go through when they realize that they are dying have been ably described by Kübler-Ross (1969). There are five stages: denial and a feeling of isolation, anger and resentment, a brief bargaining period which attempts to postpone the inevitable, depression and finally acceptance. These stages last for a variable time and may coexist or even be absent in any particular individual. The one thing that is clear, though, is that the doctor who is open and honest assists his patient towards an active acceptance of his fate. Throughout these adjustments there is, inevitably, hope. Hope that something will happen, that something will turn up to allow recovery. This hope must never be destroyed by an urge to make the patient 'face the facts'. There is no need for the doctor to lie, but he can show his patient that he keeps an open mind and can assure him that he will do everything possible to help.

Valuable practical advice is given by Twycross (1975), formerly research fellow at St. Christopher's Hospice.

(1) Do not isolate the patient.
There is an unfortunate tendency for the dying patient to be shut off in a side ward. This is partly because of a desire to give him some privacy, but sometimes reflects the embarrassment and feelings of helplessness of the ward staff who are more comfortable when the patient is out of sight, and also it may be thought kinder to spare the feelings of the other patients. Attempts to protect other patients from the sight of death are not always for the best. Particularly in residential homes the disappearance of a person, who is never spoken of again by the staff, is likely to cause considerable fear and disquiet among the remaining residents. The dying patient feels acutely lonely, and staff and relatives must be encouraged not to shy away or to treat him with false bonhomie. Sitting down with the patient instead of standing at the end of the bed imparts a sense of companionship and allows him to talk more easily if he feels like it.

(2) Communicating the truth.
Parish priests will often remark that elderly persons are very often ready and even eager to talk about death. Indeed, some patients exhausted by years of ill health welcome the release of death but are nonetheless comforted by matter-of-fact discus-

sion, particularly if the doctor reassures them that the passing will be painless. More difficult is the management of the patient who is not yet reconciled to death. Very rarely is it a case of 'shall I or shall I not tell him', but rather 'when and how shall I share this with him'. The best approach is to listen carefully for signs which indicate that the patient is ready to talk. Such remarks as 'when will I be going home?' or 'I'm not getting any better am I?' are a request for further information, and the answers should be honest yet gentle. The truth should never be forced on anyone and some patients show by their attitude that they have no wish to discuss the outcome of their illness. Cancer is an emotive word, conjuring up for most people a painful and hideous end, and if the patient uses the word it is important for the doctor to stress that pain and distressing symptoms can and will be relieved.

(3) Remembering the relatives.
Most patients, particularly if the final illness has been a long one, recognize the approach of death, although they may not talk about it. Yet very often there is a conspiracy of silence in which the relatives keep up the pretence that all will be well and avoid any mention of the subject which is of most concern to the patient. Sometimes relatives are heard making such remarks as: 'We must never tell him, it would kill him if he knew'. All too often the patient feels estranged and let down by the very people he most cherishes. The doctor should not agree to maintain a deceit and can point out that it is the patient's illness, and that if he wants to talk about it he will be encouraged to do so. It should be recognized that relatives too must pass through the five stages described by Kübler-Ross and need help in coming to terms with death.

They often welcome a chance to talk, and it is useful to enquire how they are coping at home and to allow them to unburden themselves of their fears. Many families feel guilty that their relative is dying in hospital and not at home, and need reassuring that they have done everything possible. Some

327

will want to take the patient home for the last few days and this should be encouraged.

Pain

The one thing that a doctor can virtually always guarantee his dying patient is relief of pain, yet it is all too common for this relief to be denied. The pain may not just be physical but also mental, social and spiritual, and the attack on it must be total. A report on 220 patients dying in a geriatric ward found that 13.6% complained of moderate to severe pain during their terminal illness and a further 7.7% complained of other distressing symptoms such as persistent nausea and vomiting, dysphagia and dyspnoea (Exton-Smith, 1961). Anxiety, depression and isolation will aggravate pain and must also be treated.

For mild pain paracetamol 1 g, 4-hourly or soluble aspirin 1200 mg 4-hourly are suitable. Moderate or severe pain is often relieved by the new analgesic diflunisal (Dolabid), one or two tablets 12-hourly. We have, however, found that among the very elderly there is a risk of gastric bleeding with this drug.

When the pain is severe there should be no hesitation in using morphine or diamorphine. It is important to remember that the aim is to relieve chronic pain completely. It is no good producing troughs of pain in between doses, since the patient's anxiety remains high and he is left with the unavoidable conclusion that his doctor is capable of treating his pain but chooses not to relieve it continuously. Thus opiates should never be prescribed on a p.r.n. basis, since if the patient has to ask for more analgesics the treatment is failing. Similarly it is best to avoid pethidine since it is too short-acting, lasting only about $2\frac{1}{2}$ hours. Sedation is usually undesirable in the dying patient with chronic pain, and the dose of opiate must be individually determined so as to relieve pain but not produce stupor. In moderate pain morphine 5 mg in chloroform water to 10 ml should be given orally every 4 hours and the dose adjusted upwards as necessary. A phenothiazine, prochlorperazine (Stemetil) 5 mg, is usually given in

328

addition to potentiate the morphine and because of its anti-emetic and tranquillizing effect. In severe pain morphine 20–60 mg and sometimes up to 100 mg 4-hourly will be needed. It is best to avoid the traditional cocktails (e.g. mist euphoria) since they are often too sickly and contain cocaine, which is of no benefit. The dose should always be given orally (no-one likes 4-hourly injections) unless the patient is too ill to swallow.

Dextromoramide (Palfium) 5 mg is equivalent in terms of peak effect to morphine 15 mg but acts for only 1 or 2 hours. It is therefore useful as a back-up drug, in addition to regular doses of morphine, when there is intermittent breakthrough pain. Bone pain due to metastases may be relieved by radiotherapy or by phenylbutazone, starting with 600 mg/day and reducing after a week to 300 mg/day.

There are many myths surrounding the use of morphine, but in general it can be confidently stated that addiction is not a problem when oral opiates are given for the relief of pain and that even large doses do not kill patients. Indeed it is our experience that when very ill, pain-racked patients are started on morphine they noticeably improve due to the relief of pain and anxiety.

Constipation

This is inevitable when opiates are given to an inactive patient who is not eating anything. Impacted faeces should be removed manually or with an enema, and regular doses of a laxative given, e.g. Dorbanex medo 5–10 ml twice daily.

Vomiting

The phenothiazines are often effective. Prochlorperazine (Stemetil) 5 mg orally or a 25 mg suppository causes less sedation than chlorpromazine (Largactil) 25 mg orally or a 100 mg suppository. If these fail metoclopramide (Maxolon) 10 mg orally or as an i.m. injection may be tried.

Geriatrics

Dyspnoea

Salbutamol 2–4 mg three times a day or aminophylline suppositories are used to relieve bronchospasm. Prednisolone 10–15 mg three times a day is also useful, particularly where there is widespread malignancy in the lungs. When the symptoms are severe and distressing, morphine should be given orally or diamorphine by i.m. injection.

Bronchopneumonia

The unthinking use of antibiotics may merely prolong the terminal phase and it is often better to give a small dose of morphine to relieve distress, a tranquillizer to ease anxiety and atropine 0.6 mg i.m. to dry up troublesome secretions. If the patient complains of a dry mouth he should be given ice to suck, or frequent small drinks. Intravenous fluids or a nasogastric tube are rarely indicated.

REFERENCES

Exton-Smith, A. N. (1961). Terminal illness in the aged. *Lancet*, **ii**, 305
Illich, I. (1975). *Medical Nemesis*. (London: Calder & Boyars)
Kübler-Ross, E. (1969). *On Death and Dying*. (New York: Macmillan)
Twycross, R. G. (1975). *The Dying Patient*. (London: Christian Medical Fellowship)

Index